Food Allergies

Enjoying Life with a Severe Food Allergy

Tanya Wright, BSc (Hons), SRD

State Registered Dietitian, working at Stoke Mandeville Hospital as Head of the Nutrition and Dietetic Department. She runs the Allergy Support Group, is a Regional Coordinator for the Anaphylaxis Campaign and for the British Allergy Foundation and is on the Medical Board of the British Allergy Foundation.

Medical adviser: **Dr Joanne Clough** DM, FRCA, MRCP, FRCPCH

Senior Lecturer in Paediatric Respiratory Medicine at Southampton General Hospital, and a member of the British Society of Allergy and Clinical Immunology. She runs a clinic for children with allergies.

CLASS PUBLISHING · LONDON

Printing history
First published 2001

The author and publishers welcome feedback from the users of this book.
Please contact the publishers.

Class Publishing, Barb House, Barb Mews, London W6 7PA, UK
Telephone: (020) 7371 2119
Fax: (020) 7371 2878

Email: post@class.co.uk

Website: http//www.class.co.uk

A CIP catalogue record for this book is available from the British Library

ISBN 1 85959 039 X

The information presented in this book is accurate and current to the best
of the author's knowledge. The author and publisher, however, make no
guarantee as to, and assume no responsibility for, the correctness, sufficiency
or completeness of such information or recommendation. The reader is
advised to consult a doctor regarding all aspects of individual health care.

Edited by Gillian Clarke

Designed and typeset by Martin Bristow

Index by Valerie Elliston

Printed and bound in Finland by WS Bookwell, Juva

Contents

ENJOYING FOOD

ENJOYING LIFE

Foreword

by **David Reading**
Director, The Anaphylaxis Campaign

Food allergy has become big news during the last decade. Rarely does a week go by without a dramatic story appearing in the newspapers or on TV. Peanut allergy, in particular, has become a source of sensational news reports and often the reader is left in no doubt that allergies can be serious. On rare occasions they kill.

Yet the help available for the food allergic patient is often appallingly inadequate. It depends to some extent on where you live. Many doctors in general practice or running allergy clinics provide a wealth of vital information and practical guidance. But all too often, patients emerge from their consultation feeling totally despondent and unprepared to face the challenges ahead. The burden that families face is often overwhelming, particularly if it is a child who has a potentially severe food allergy.

As a founder member of the Anaphylaxis Campaign – a national charity set up in 1994 to help people manage their allergies – I became aware from the outset of the huge gaps in information available. Every day, we receive urgent appeals for help: What can I do to educate my child's school? Can I trust food labels? What do the results of my allergy tests mean?

Thankfully, there are people around who have made it their business to investigate the problems of food allergy, identify solutions and pass on their knowledge to others. Tanya Wright, the author of this book, has lived with severe milk allergy for eight years, and during that time has encountered most of the pitfalls. She has learned crucial lessons the hard way, and developed the message that it is perfectly possible to enjoy life with a severe food allergy so long as you are well equipped with information.

A huge amount of that information is presented in this book, making it an indispensable guide. Bon appetit!

Foreword

by **Maureen Jenkins**
Nurse Adviser and Training Coordinator, British Allergy Foundation

Along with asthma, rhinitis and eczema, the incidence of food allergy is rising alarmingly. At present, between 1.4% and 1.9% of the adult population have a true food allergy, and about 5% of young children. The severity may vary between individuals but always affects the quality of life of both the people with food allergies and their families or carers, involving constantly monitoring of the ingredients – often 'hidden' – of everything that is consumed. Some of the foods causing these potentially life-threatening reactions are those most commonly consumed or frequently used in food manufacture.

The inadequate number of NHS allergy clinics usually means a very long wait for an appointment with an allergy specialist. Even when the allergy has been diagnosed, many allergy clinics have little or no access to specialist dietitians to guide the person through the minefield that is ahead. Most people with food allergies rely on advice from specialist medical charities and from others with the same problem.

Although there are now many books about food intolerance, very little has been produced to help those with true food allergy. Tanya Wright has amalgamated her personal experience of severe food allergy with her expertise as a specialist dietitian, to produce this unsurpassed guide to living with food allergy. Everything about allergic disease is simply but comprehensively explained, including coping with anaphylaxis. The intricacies of referral for diagnosis, foreign travel, career and leisure choices, and information about help from other agencies are all thoroughly covered. A large section is devoted to practical help with special diets, including alternative foods and the names and addresses of specialist food manufacturers. I challenge anyone to find a question about the subject of severe food allergy that is unanswered in this wonderful book.

Author's note

The purpose of writing this book was to bring together both my professional and my personal experience of living life with a severe food allergy. It is aimed at people with a severe food allergy and their families, and the healthcare workers dealing with them, to provide a useful resource as well as a source of comfort for those who are anxious about living with their condition.

Reading this book and using the relevant information should help you to *Enjoy Life with a Severe Food Allergy!*

Acknowledgements

We are very grateful to the many people who have helped in the development of this book. In particular, we thank:

Dr Joanne Clough, for allowing us to use some Glossary entries from her book *Allergies at your fingertips*

and for their reviews of the manuscript:
Marianne de Giorgio, mother of children with food allergies
Lorna Downing, mother in a family with food allergies
Arthur Ling, Managing Director of Plamil Foods
Dr Anna Moore, MBBS, DipNutritional Medicine, a GP with special interest in nutrition
David Reading, Director of The Anaphylaxis Campaign
Grieg Saunders, Product Manager at Provamel
Muriel Simmons, Chief Executive of the British Allergy Foundation, and **Maureen Jenkins**, also of the British Allergy Foundation
Christopher Swire, of Fayrefield Foods Ltd
Victoria Wick, Product Manager at Matthews Foods

About the author

Tanya Wright is a State Registered Dietitian and works at Stoke Mandeville Hospital as Head of Nutrition and Dietetic Services. She became interested in allergy because she has a severe allergy to milk and eggs and their derivatives.

In 1994 she started up an allergy support group, which she runs in her own time from the hospital. The number of queries and letters she receives continues to increase. She is also a consultant for companies making foods for special diets, is a website dietitian specialising in food allergy and has been involved with several recipe and information books for people with special diets.

Tanya is a Regional Coordinator for the Anaphylaxis Campaign and for the British Allergy Foundation, and is on the Medical Board of the British Allergy Foundation. She often gives lectures and talks as well as writing in several well-known publications on the subject of food-induced anaphylaxis.

Tanya is working on her Master's degree in 'The Mechanisms of Allergic Disease' at Southampton University, which will qualify her to undertake further roles in the field of allergy.

Introduction

The fact that you are reading this book suggests that either you or someone in your family (or perhaps both) has an allergy or intolerance to certain types of food. At a relatively minor level, eating the 'wrong' food can bring you out in a rash (hives). At an extreme level, eating even a minute amount of a trigger food can cause a very serious reaction – anaphylaxis. (Anaphylaxis can also be caused by a bee or wasp sting or a drug or latex products but in this book we will be talking only about food allergy.)

Anaphylaxis can be life-threatening, and people at risk of this severe reaction carry adrenaline with them to use in such an emergency. It seems to have become more common in recent years, and will probably continue to increase.

A number of well-publicised deaths caused by food-induced anaphylaxis have highlighted the fact that preventive measures as well as prompt treatment have an essential part to play in living with this life-threatening condition. Most cases are triggered by food eaten outside the home. In fact, most of the deaths due to food-induced anaphylaxis have resulted from food eaten in restaurants, cafés and other busy commercial eating-places.

Media coverage and pressure groups such as the Anaphylaxis Campaign have greatly increased awareness of the practical problems of living with the threat of anaphylaxis. The Ministry of Agriculture Fisheries and Foods (MAFF) and the Food Standards Agency are working with the food industry, health professionals and consumer groups to help address these problems. Food manufacturers and retailers and the food and catering industries are making many positive changes to their practices and labelling to minimise the risks of susceptible people ingesting foods to which they are allergic.

The information in this book will complement the work that is taking place by enabling you to be more proactive in preventing severe reactions to food. If an allergic reaction does occur, having a plan of action and all the necessary treatment to hand is the foundation of successful management. Even if you are not at risk of an anaphylactic reaction, the information here will help you to live a normal life despite having to avoid certain foods or ingredients.

Background

1
Food Allergy

WHAT IS ALLERGY?

An allergy is an inappropriate and harmful response of the body's defence mechanisms to substances that are normally harmless. Allergic reactions involve the immune system, which protects us from infections by viruses, bacteria and parasites. When a potentially harmful attacker, such as the measles virus or a staphylococcus bacterium, invades our body, the many different parts of the immune system work together, signalling to one another using chemical messengers, to surround and kill the attacker before serious damage is done. The first time the body encounters a new type of germ, it will be several days before the infection is overcome. However, the immune system retains a memory of the attacker, so that future infections are dealt with promptly and efficiently. This memory is in the form of *antibodies*, which are small proteins that are tailor-made for each attacker. There are several different types of antibody, and the main ones involved in fighting infections are immunoglobulin A (IgA), immunoglobulin M (IgM) and immunoglobulin E (IgE).

In people who develop allergies, the immune system works perfectly well against infectious organisms. In addition, though, it has a tendency to react to normally harmless substances as if they were attackers. When this happens, the immune system becomes *sensitised* to the substance – it mistakenly identifies the substance as a hostile factor and, by producing antibodies against it, programmes the body to react whenever it is encountered. Whenever the body encounters this substance again, an allergic reaction results. Substances that cause this reaction are known as *allergens*, which are almost always protein molecules. When the body encounters an allergen, even in tiny amounts, large quantities of allergy antibodies (immunoglobulin E, or IgE) are made, which react with the allergen to set off a series of events called the *allergic reaction*. This process involves many different parts of the immune system, co-ordinated by chemical messengers released by the white blood cells.

5

Most of the damage to the body's tissues that occurs during an allergic reaction is a result of the release of the chemicals from a type of cell called the *mast cell*. Mast cells are one of the cells that make up the immune system and are found in many different tissues of the body. (They are particularly common in the airways of the lung, in the bowel wall, and in the eyes, nose and throat.) These chemicals are stored inside the mast cell in tiny packages, or granules. When an allergen reacts with the IgE antibodies on the surface of the mast cell, these granules are released. The chemicals in them have a number of effects, including the enlargement of small blood vessels, increased leakiness of the blood vessel walls, the contraction of the muscle in the bowel wall and lung airways, and the increased secretion of mucus. These changes lead to the redness, tenderness and swelling commonly known as inflammation.

This allergic inflammation has different effects in different parts of the body. In the lungs it causes coughing and wheezing – the symptoms of asthma. In the nose it causes runniness and blockage – the symptoms of rhinitis or hay-fever. In the bowel it causes colicky pain and diarrhoea, or, in the mouth, itching and tingling – the symptoms of food allergy. Sometimes the allergic reaction involves the skin, leading to itching and skin rashes.

WHO CAN DEVELOP ALLERGIES?

People whose parents or other close relatives have allergic disease have a greater tendency than others to develop an allergy at some time in their lives. The most common allergic diseases are asthma, eczema and hay-fever. The tendency to develop an allergy, known as *atopy* (from the Greek 'atopia', meaning 'out of place'), seems therefore to be inherited. Atopic individuals are much more likely to develop allergic disease if they are exposed to certain environmental factors or *triggers*.

HOW COMMON IS ALLERGY?

The number of people affected by allergy has increased dramatically since the early 1970s, particularly in developed countries, and it continues to increase. Allergies now affect up to one-third of the population in industrialised countries. It is predicted that, as Third World countries develop, a similar pattern will develop there. The

World Health Organization has labelled allergy 'the number one environmental disease'.

In the UK, as many as one person in three will experience at least one form of allergic disease during their lifetime. Although as many as 20% of the population believe that they are allergic to one or more foods, in reality only about 2–3% have true food allergy. In others, the adverse reactions to food may be due to a different, non-allergenic, mechanism. Allergy is more common in children under three years of age, in whom it occurs in about 10%. It is thought that this difference is related to the development of the body's immune system – it is still developing in young children.

The foods responsible for the vast majority of food-induced reactions are milk, eggs, peanuts, tree nuts, shellfish and fish.

WHY ARE ALLERGIES INCREASING?

A number of environmental factors may increase people's susceptibility to allergy. They include modern housing, the Western diet, family size and the over-use of antibiotics.

Housing

As a result of double glazing, good insulation and efficient heating systems, the humidity and temperature of our homes and work/social environments have risen to levels that encourage high numbers of house dust mites, whose faecal droppings contain an allergen. This, plus an increase in the use of soft furnishings (carpets, curtains, cushions) in which the house dust mite thrives and the growing popularity of pets, means an increase in allergen levels. The effect is increased because people now tend to spend more time indoors.

Diet

There is some evidence to indicate that changes in our diet also play a part. Whereas 30–40 years ago most food was fresh, nowadays much of it is processed and contains many additives. Moreover, processed foods contain fewer natural antioxidants and vitamins, which are abundant in fresh fruit and vegetables, and which are thought to protect against a number of conditions – including allergic diseases.

Family size and childhood infections

Children from smaller families seem to be more likely to develop an allergy. This is thought to be because they are exposed to fewer viral infections in early life than children in larger families. This applies especially to those who have not attended nursery or playgroup. Frequent infections in early life promote a switch to the non-allergic state as opposed to the allergic state, which makes it much less likely that an individual will develop an allergic condition in later life.

Antibiotics
The increasing use of antibiotics in early life (and their inclusion in foodstuffs via animal feed) may alter the balance of the 'friendly' germs found on the skin and in the bowel. This may, in turn, increase the risk of developing allergic diseases.

ADVERSE REACTIONS TO FOODS

There are many different ways in which our bodies can react adversely to foodstuffs. Some of these are predictable and will occur in everybody to a greater or lesser extent. They include the effects of foodstuffs such as those containing caffeine or alcohol, and the

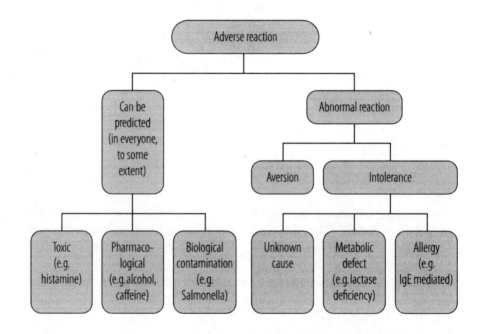

Figure 1.1 Types of adverse reactions to food

results of eating food contaminated with micro-organisms such as salmonella, which causes food poisoning. All other adverse reactions to food are abnormal in that they do not occur in everyone, just in certain individuals. These reactions include *food aversion*, a psychological reaction that occurs only when the person knows that they have eaten a particular food, and *food intolerance*, when there is a genuine and repeatable reaction to a particular food.

There are two main types of food intolerance. In *metabolic defects* individuals have abnormally low levels of the enzymes that digest certain foods, and so they are unable to tolerate those foods (e.g. lactose intolerance). The other main form of food intolerance is *food allergy*, which occurs when an individual's immune system has become sensitised to a particular allergen, which then subsequently causes allergic reactions – for example, hives (urticaria) or swelling of the face, lips and tongue (angio-oedema). Figure 1.1 places food allergy in context with other adverse reactions to food.

Anaphylaxis is the most extreme reaction of a food allergy, and is discussed in Chapter 4.

What happens during an allergic reaction?

An allergic reaction to food can cause a range of symptoms in a number of different parts of the body:

- swelling of the lips, tongue and face (angio-oedema),
- itchy 'nettle' rash on the trunk and limbs (urticaria/hives),
- wheezing and shortness of breath,
- runny nose and inflamed eyes (rhino-conjunctivitis),
- swelling of the voicebox (the larynx),
- colicky abdominal pain, nausea and vomiting,
- life-threatening collapse with shock (anaphylaxis),

as well as flushing, palpitations, feelings of anxiety and faintness.

All these reactions are caused by immune responses involving IgE antibodies. They occur very quickly after the allergen has been ingested – within minutes. Occasionally, other symptoms can come on after a delay of a few hours; these include abdominal pain, diarrhoea and a worsening of eczema. The most common foods that cause food allergy in the UK are cow's milk, hen's eggs, peanuts, tree nuts, fish and shellfish.

There are several other types of 'immune-mediated adverse food reactions' that do not involve IgE. They include coeliac disease, which is an intolerance of the protein called gluten, found in wheat, rye, oats and barley.

TREATMENT

How severe reactions are treated is discussed in Chapter 4. The treatment of less severe reactions will depend on the symptoms, and may involve avoiding specific food (or foods), or taking antihistamines or any of a variety of therapies specific to the individual's symptoms. Exclusion diets are useful in identifying food intolerances and less severe food allergies. They are discussed in Chapter 8 ('The Dietitian's Role').

SUMMARY

You should now understand more about what happens during an allergic reaction. Later in this book you will find out about the different types of food allergies and their management.

2
Food Allergy Tests

Allergy testing carried out by your GP or at an allergy clinic will help to identify which substances you are allergic to. But the appropriate tests can only be chosen when the details of your medical history have been considered. Unfortunately, no allergy test will predict the nature and severity of your reactions in the future.

WHAT TO DO IF YOU THINK YOU HAVE A FOOD ALLERGY

You may suspect you have a food allergy, for a number of reasons, and you may also feel that you know what the offending food is. However, to be sure of the exact nature of the allergy and for the correct treatment to be prescribed, the allergens should be identified by your doctor using safe and accurate methods.

Before you keep your appointment with your GP or the allergy specialist, note down as much information as possible about your symptoms. You can use the following checklist as a guide to the sort of information to keep:

- Your symptoms: what, where, when, for how long?
- The exact circumstances leading the symptoms; for example:
  - what had you eaten?
  - how long after you ate it did symptoms begin?
  - where had you eaten it?
  - were there other foods around at the time?
  - who had prepared the food?
- Your own and your family history of atopy (asthma, eczema, hay-fever, food allergies, anaphylaxis).
- Foods you think may have caused the symptoms.
- Other factors that might have caused the reaction.
- Frequency of the reactions.
- Details of past reactions.
- Details of medication taken following a severe reaction.

Keeping a record of these facts will help the doctor to diagnose your problem and, if it is due to allergy, to identify the allergens. Even if you know what is causing your reaction, it is still important to go through this process for confirmation to ensure that an allergy is indeed the problem and, if so, to check for any cross-reactivity and to see if you are allergic to any other allergens. With cross-reactivity, two or more allergens induce similar reactions. The allergens may be from the same food group or from different food groups (see Chapter 12, 'Cross-reactivity and Food Families').

DIAGNOSIS OF A FOOD ALLERGY

Diagnosing a food allergy and identifying the offending foods is done largely on the basis of your medical history but may also require allergy testing. These tests should be performed and interpreted by a practitioner with the appropriate training and experience, because no test is 100% reliable. All results should be considered in relation to your history and symptoms.

A diagnosis of food allergy can be made if there is:

- a positive medical history plus a positive skin-prick or RAST test (see below),
- a positive medical history plus a positive response to a 'food challenge' in which neither you nor the person doing the testing knows what the food being tested actually is (a double-blind food challenge),
- a positive medical history plus a positive objective response to 'open challenge' (i.e. both you and the person doing the testing know what foods you are being given) such as symptoms or a change in the cellular structure (histology) of the lining of the small bowel.

Diagnosing yourself (self-diagnosis) is inadvisable. If, for example, you cut too many foods out of your diet without adequate nutritional replacement, you may do more harm than good. For this reason it is essential to obtain recognised professional help when trying to detect food allergies. Once a food allergy has been diagnosed you may then be referred to a state registered dietitian, who will give you detailed advice on which foods to avoid and how to replace them with suitable alternatives so that you can maintain a nutritionally balanced diet (see Chapter 8, 'The Dietitian's Role').

TESTING FOR A SUSPECTED FOOD ALLERGY

Once a food allergy is suspected, one or more of the following tests may be done to confirm the diagnosis. Usually the simplest tests are done first.

Skin-prick test (SPT)

This is the most commonly used, fastest and easiest way to detect an allergy. The basis of a skin-prick test is that it demonstrates the presence of allergen-specific immunoglobulin E (IgE) attached to the skin's mast cells (see Chapter 1). It involves placing a liquid extract of the suspected allergen on the skin (usually the forearm) and pricking the skin through it so as to just puncture the skin, without drawing blood. If there is a positive reaction to the sample allergen, a small bump (called a weal) will come up, reaching its maximum size within 15–20 minutes. It looks quite like nettle rash, and is likely to be red and itchy. The reaction disappears within an hour.

Anything from one to 25 allergens can be tested at a time, although it is more usual to test only three to six. Each area of the skin that is being tested is marked with a pen, so that the reaction can be identified later. The amount of allergen introduced into the skin is so tiny that a serious reaction is extremely unlikely, even in someone who has previously had an anaphylactic reaction to that substance. In addition to the allergens to be tested, positive and negative 'controls' are used to ensure that the test is being performed correctly.

The **negative control** is a saline (salt water) solution, to which no response is expected. If there is a response, it may be that the skin is over-sensitive to pressure and that the response to the test is a 'false positive'. If this happens, the doctor will interpret the results with the utmost care, and may even decide that the whole test is invalid.

The **positive control** is a solution containing a standard concentration of histamine, to which everyone is expected to react. If there is no response to the positive control solution, it is possible that something is preventing the skin from developing an allergic reaction. A number of drugs can do this, including all antihistamine preparations, some antidepressants, some cough mixtures and, under certain conditions, preparations that contain steroids. These medications should, if possible, be stopped before the skin testing. If you are waiting to see the GP or allergy specialist for an initial appointment, it may be useful to contact them to find out when you need to stop your medication.

Times vary between two days and about one month.

It is possible to have an unexpectedly positive result to a skin-prick test that does not fit in with your medical history. This is known as a *false positive response*. There are several reasons for a false positive skin test. For example:

- An allergy may be developing to a food but you have not yet experienced an allergic reaction – 'latent allergy'.
- The food extract used in the test is not identical to the actual food that you eat.
- The allergen may be prepared differently from when it is used in food (e.g. raw rather than cooked).
- The allergen extract may have been contaminated with a substance to which you do react.
- The wrong test site has been used (different parts of the skin react differently).
- The test has been administered improperly.
- The person being tested is very young or very old

A *false negative result* might be obtained if:

- the person being tested has recently had a severe allergic reaction (it takes about three to four weeks for the levels of IgE in the body to return to normal),
- the extract used is of poor quality or is out of date.

These problems are relatively uncommon, and the skin-prick test is a useful tool in the diagnosis of a food allergy. It is, however, important that a doctor experienced in this field interprets the test results.

Blood test – radio-allergosorbent test (RAST)

For this, a small sample of your blood will be taken from a vein in your arm and sent to the local hospital laboratory for testing. The results – which are usually available in 7 to 14 days – are a measure of the amount of IgE produced in response to individual allergens. Results are graded according to the strength of the reaction. Blood tests are not affected by antihistamines, so they can be used with people who have severe eczema.

RAST tests are relatively expensive, so should be used in conjunction with other tests such as skin-prick testing. Examples of when this blood test is indicated include:

- in the very young, in whom skin testing can be unreliable,
- in people with extensive skin lesions (e.g. eczema), in whom skin testing is difficult,
- if solutions of the relevant allergen are not suitable to go on the skin,
- in people who are unable to stop taking their antihistamine medication,
- where skin-prick tests are unavailable.

The results of RAST tests are classified from 0 (negative) rising to 4 or 6 (extremely high) – the scale used will depend on the hospital. For example:

Class	Level of sensitivity to the tested allergen
0	Negative
1	Low
2	Moderate
3	High
4	Extremely high

As with skin-prick tests, it is possible to get false negative and false positive results with RAST tests. For this reason and because the range of allergens available for testing is not fully comprehensive, the results of these 'assays' should not be viewed alone, without knowledge of the person's medical history and food and symptom diaries (see below). The CAP-RAST test seems to be taking over from the RAST test because it appears to be more reliable and more sensitive.

Blood test for coeliac disease

There is now a blood test that can give a general indication that a person probably has coeliac disease – a serious but not life-threatening condition. To be sure, though, a gastroscopy has to be done. This involves putting a tube down into the person's gut to remove a sample of tissue. This biopsy will show whether or not the condition is present.

Food challenge test

There are two types of 'food challenge':

- **Open food challenge** You are given increasing quantities of the food to which it is thought you are allergic and your symptoms are noted. In this test both you and the doctor administering the food know what it is.
- **Double-blind placebo-controlled food challenge** Both the food in question and a harmless dummy (the placebo) are encased in gelatine capsules and given in random order so that neither you nor the doctor knows which food (if any) is being taken. This is important because sometimes an unpleasant reaction to food can occur because of psychological associations; for example, if you have previously been very ill after eating seafood, just the sight of seafood might make you feel sick.

A food challenge is likely to be offered when:

- there is uncertainty as to whether a food allergy exists,
- the doctor wishes to find out if an allergy has been outgrown (after having confirmed that the result of skin-prick or RAST testing is negative),
- confirmation of a suspected allergy is required,
- a food is to be taken for the first time (e.g. when a food has been avoided for many years because of a history of allergy in the family).

This test will be performed in hospital – either in the outpatient department or in a ward – by a person trained in the management of severe allergic reactions. This is because there is a small chance that a severe reaction might occur.

Sequential food challenge

The foods or ingredients to be tested will be given in a set order – sequential food challenge. For example, first milk and milk products, followed by egg and egg products followed by yeast, and then wheat. If egg is being tested, the yolk of a hard-boiled egg will be tried and then the white. But, as with all other tests, this must be done under the supervision of a medical professional. *Never* try to do this on your own.

The food/symptom diary

A food/symptom diary can be very useful in determining which foods cause an allergic reaction. Every day you note down everything you eat and drink, giving the date and time, and then record the time and details of any symptoms you experience. The diary might be kept for just a few days or for longer periods, as necessary. The information gained will:

- show how you are normally,
- assess any symptoms when you exclude certain foods from your diet,
- assess any symptoms when you reintroduce certain foods into your diet.

Dietary manipulation

There are a variety of 'dietary manipulation' methods that can be used in the diagnosis of a food allergy: they are exclusion, elimination and few-foods diets. Details of these can be found in Chapter 8 ('The Dietitian's Role').

A combination of your allergic/medical history, food and symptom records, suspect foods and the results from these three diets may help in making a diagnosis of food allergy. The method used will be specific to your individual needs. Skin-prick and RAST tests can be used as indicators of food allergy. Their results can help determine which foods to incorporate in a trial exclusion diet and in which order foods should be reintroduced (challenged) into the diet.

Once food allergens have been identified successfully, it is generally necessary to completely avoid the offending food(s) and any components or derivatives of these foods. To do this successfully usually requires the help of a dietitian (see Chapter 8), who will advise on avoiding food(s) and replacing them with substitutes of similar nutritional quality. If, though, the allergy is only a mild intolerance, it is not always necessary to avoid the food completely – it may be tolerated in small amounts (e.g. someone with lactose intolerance may be able to tolerate up to a cup of milk a day).

FACTORS THAT MAY AFFECT THE ALLERGIC RESPONSE

Several factors may trigger an allergic response:

- exercise,
- infection,
- alcohol,
- medication.

These are discussed in Chapter 4 ('Anaphylaxis').

COMPLEMENTARY THERAPIES

Complementary medicine practitioners and their skills have a lot to offer and they can provide very effective therapies for *some* conditions. However, there are many 'alternative' allergy tests on offer that are *not* regarded by conventional practitioners to be relevant and are considered to have no place in the diagnosis of true allergy. These include kinesiology, hair analysis, pulse test, sublingual provocation test, urine test, sweat test, radionics and vega testing, to name a few. They may be offered through supermarkets, healthfood shops, health farms, newspapers, the *Yellow Pages* and glossy magazines.

The drawbacks of having such tests are:

- the method of testing is inappropriate for severe food allergy,
- the resulting diagnosis may be inaccurate,
- inappropriate and unbalanced diets may be recommended,
- it is often suggested that a large number of foods are avoided for an indefinite period of time, with little or no adequate dietetic review,
- failure to recognise and treat a genuine disease,
- they are often undertaken by medically unqualified staff,
- the creation of fictitious disease entities.

Any of these can lead to malnutrition and disturbed growth in children, unintentional weight loss, food phobias, frustration and anger when things do not improve, disruption of one's lifestyle and a poor quality of life.

FOLLOWING THE DIAGNOSIS OF A FOOD ALLERGY

If you are diagnosed as having a food allergy you will probably be referred to a dietitian, who will give you advice about the foods and ingredients that you can eat safely and devise a management plan. For a severe food allergy this will involve:

- total exclusion of the offending food from your diet,
- making sure that you fully understand the new diet and are able to follow it,
- arranging for follow-up appointments from time to time as long as you need them, to deal with any problems or questions,
- any medication that you should carry with you at all times,
- a plan of action to be followed (including emergency treatment) if you are accidentally exposed to the offending food (see Chapter 5, 'Your Anaphylaxis Contingency Plan').

If your child has been diagnosed as having a severe food allergy, it will be important to make sure that friends, playmates and school staff also understand all about it. Liaising with your child's school is dealt with in Chapter 6 ('Anaphylaxis and Going to School').

The role of the dietitian is discussed more fully in Chapter 8.

TESTING FOR LATEX ALLERGY

Allergy to certain foods may be related to an allergy to latex ('cross-reactivity', discussed in Chapter 12). It can take from 20 minutes to 48 hours for a reaction to occur. A suspected latex allergy can be tested by a number of methods, including a patch test, a skin-prick test or a RAST test.

A positive result to any of these tests means that efforts must be made to avoid any contact with latex. If you are in hospital or at the dentist, it is essential that you ask for non-latex examination gloves to be used. This is particularly important if the procedure is to happen under a general anaesthetic, as you will not be awake to remind the staff at the last minute when the gloves come out!

REFERRAL TO AN ALLERGY SPECIALIST

If you have, or suspect that you have, an allergy, the first port of call is usually your general practitioner (GP). If your GP feels that further investigation is required, you may be referred to a specialist in allergies. Allergy specialists are usually part of an NHS hospital-based allergy clinic, and their services can be accessed only by referral from either a GP or a hospital doctor. Self-referral is not an option in the UK.

Obtaining a referral from the GP is not always straightforward. Sometimes people feel that they should have been referred to an allergy clinic but their GP did not sanction it. This is often because the GP had the necessary skills required to give the advice. Most allergy services in the UK are provided by GPs, paediatricians (children's doctors), chest or respiratory physicians (e.g. for asthma), dermatologists (for skin problems, such as eczema) and doctors specialising in ear, nose and throat (ENT) conditions (such as rhinitis). Specialists in an allergy clinic generally tend to see the very young, people with very severe food allergy or with multiple food allergies and people with undiagnosed problems that might be due to an allergy.

Another possibility for non-referral might be that the GP was unaware of the availability of this service and how to locate it. So polite persistence may be needed. Some people seek a second opinion from another GP. In the rare occasions that a person is still unhappy about their treatment, a possible option is to contact the local community health council (CHC). This is an independent body with a voice on health issues in the community, which helps individuals who are dissatisfied with the health care that they have received. (The address and telephone number are in the local telephone directory.)

GPs who wish to locate their nearest NHS allergy clinic can consult the *National Health Service Allergy Clinics Handbook* (see Appendix 2, 'Useful Publications'), which provides information on allergy services in the UK. Allergy is a very broad subject and the services provided by allergy clinics can vary enormously, so this handbook is designed to provide GPs and referring doctors with detailed information about each clinic, so that they can refer appropriately.

The doctors in NHS allergy clinics should be members of the British Society for Allergy and Clinical Immunology (BSACI), which regulates the standards of care in such clinics. They should also follow the Code of Good Allergy Practice, outlined in the *Standards of Care for Providers of Allergy Services within the NHS*, supported by the

BSACI and the British Allergy Foundation (BAF). Details of allergy clinics listed in the *National Health Service Allergy Clinics Handbook* are available from the British Allergy Foundation, the Anaphylaxis Campaign or direct from the BSACI (see Appendix 1) but they are unable to give names of individual consultants.

Unfortunately, there are very few NHS allergy clinics in the UK to cope with the increasing number of people with severe allergies, which is why there are often long waiting lists. The allergy clinics that do exist are not evenly spread geographically, which may mean people having to travel a long distance to the one most appropriate for them.

A study published in 1999 by the BSACI (the professional body for doctors working in allergy) reported that the UK has only five NHS clinics offering a full-time multi-disciplinary allergy service, with a further 115 providing only part-time services. These figures equate to only one full-time allergist for every 2.1 million population. There have been various campaigns to raise awareness of the inadequate provision. The Royal College of Physicians has responded by providing more opportunities for doctors to train in the field of allergy, and services are now gradually increasing.

In May 1994, the government's Chief Medical Officer issued clear guidelines to GPs regarding the referral of patients with suspected peanut allergy for specialist advice. Although the report – Chief Medical Officer's Update 2 'Peanut anaphylaxis' – deals specifically with peanut allergy, the guidelines are also appropriate when dealing with potentially severe symptoms caused by allergy to other foods and non-food substances, including sesame, milk, eggs, fish, shellfish, certain medications and latex. GPs should be aware of the contents of this report. The Anaphylaxis Campaign (contact details in Appendix 1) has a factsheet about it.

3

Will My Allergy Improve over Time?

People with a severe food allergy often ask about the likelihood of growing out of it or, if this is not possible, if there are alternatives to living with it, such as an allergy vaccine or a medical treatment. This chapter discusses the possibilities.

DESENSITISATION AND IMMUNOTHERAPY

Immunotherapy (also known as 'desensitisation') is a well-established treatment for certain allergies caused by allergens that are inhaled – for example, for pollen and house dust mite – but *not* for foods. Starting with a minute dose, increasing doses of an allergen are administered until you can tolerate exposure to it without developing major symptoms. Controlled studies have demonstrated the effectiveness of immunotherapy in allergic rhinitis (hay-fever), conjunctivitis (itchy eyes), allergy-related wheeze (with or without cough), hypersensitivity to insect stings and allergies to cat dander and house dust mite.

Attempts to desensitise or immunise the body against allergens date from the 1890s. Present methods include 'enzyme-potentiated desensitisation' (EPD) and 'neutralisation' (they are not usually available on the NHS.) They are safe and effective against nearly all allergens but *only* if the reactions to them are mild. There is usually *no* place for immunotherapy in people with severe allergies because even tiny amounts of an allergen can trigger a reaction. Desensitisation is not generally used for people with multiple allergies or in those with severe asthma.

Enzyme-potentiated desensitisation (EPD)

EPD was developed in England in 1966 by Dr Leonard McEwan. It is used throughout the world, although it is not generally accepted by mainstream medicine. In the UK there are fewer than 20 private doctors who offer EPD; it is available through the NHS in two London hospitals: the Middlesex Hospital allergy clinic and the Royal London Homoeopathic Hospital. The treatment involves administering the allergen into the skin, by an injection or the scratch method, at intervals of ten weeks for about a year, every three months for the second year and every six months after that, as required. The strength of the dose given remains constant throughout. The theory is that the body gets used to and is able to tolerate previously harmful allergen(s).

Neutralisation

Neutralisation was developed in the USA by Dr J B Miller in the 1960s. Like EPD, it is now used world-wide although it is not generally accepted by mainstream medicine. The treatment consists of known or suspected allergens being diluted many times over and then injected into the arm. The dilutions injected get weaker over a period of time. The dilution that produces no reaction is the 'neutralisation point'. This dilution is the treatment dose that is then prepared and given to the person for self-administration.

Neutralisation therapy can be given in two ways: by an injection every two to three days or by drops under the tongue every four hours. Treatment should continue for two to three years to achieve long-term benefit.

In the UK there are about 15 private doctors offering neutralisation. For the names of these specialists, contact Action Against Allergy (details in Appendix 1).

VACCINE

A lot of research work is investigating the possibility of vaccine therapies for food allergy. There are two types: 'non-specific' therapies, which reduce allergic symptoms to everything to which a person is allergic; and 'specific' therapies, which reduce symptoms to individual allergens to which the therapy is directed (e.g. Brazil nut allergy). Researchers are evaluating these two approaches to block food allergy reactions.

Current research projects to develop a vaccine to peanuts include work at the Johns Hopkins University School of Medicine in Baltimore (USA) using DNA from peanuts.

GROWING OUT OF IT

Whether or not you will 'grow out of' your allergy will depend to a large extent on your age and your family history. Babies often outgrow moderate or mild food allergies, usually before they are three years old but possibly later. However, the longer they have the allergies or intolerances and the stronger the family history, the less likelihood of their outgrowing them. If you develop an allergy in adulthood, it is unlikely to disappear completely but may improve (although it might become worse) with time.

4
Anaphylaxis

The word phylaxis is the Greek for 'protection', so anaphylaxis is the opposite to this. Also known as anaphylactic shock, anaphylaxis is the most severe form of allergic reaction. It is a medical emergency characterised by shortness of breath, low blood pressure and collapse of the circulatory system carrying blood to the various organs. In extreme cases it is potentially life-threatening.

Although there is a wide range of symptoms that can occur in anaphylaxis, not all of them will be experienced on each occasion.

WHAT ARE THE CAUSES OF ANAPHYLAXIS?

Anaphylaxis, or an anaphylactic reaction, can have any of several causes, outlined below.

Certain foods Any food can cause anaphylaxis but the most likely culprits are nuts, peanuts, sesame seeds, fish, shellfish, cow's milk and eggs.

Exercise-induced anaphylaxis This usually arises only after eating a particular food – which acts as a sensitising agent – just before exercise. This type of anaphylaxis is therefore known as *food-dependent exercise-induced anaphylaxis*. Some susceptible people may be able to tolerate exercise or to eat a certain food with only a mild reaction or no reaction at all. However, exercise soon after ingesting this food causes an anaphylactic reaction. Finding out which food is having this effect may require allergy tests, and referral to an allergy clinic is essential.

Idiopathic Anaphylaxis that has no known cause, even after extensive testing, is known as idiopathic anaphylaxis.

Insect stings Every year in the UK there are between two and nine deaths from bee and wasp stings; hornets are another common cause of insect allergy. The risk of being stung can be minimised by taking precautions as outlined in the factsheet produced by the Anaphylaxis Campaign (address in Appendix 1).

Latex Gloves, condoms, balloons, elastic bands, rubber-soled shoes and many more items that are made from natural rubber latex can provoke a life-threatening allergic reaction. Latex allergy can also be associated with an allergy to certain foods; this 'cross-reactivity' is discussed in Chapter 12.

Medicines In susceptible individuals some medicines can cause anaphylaxis. Common examples are drugs containing salicylate (e.g. aspirin) and certain anaesthetics, but most drugs have the potential to cause an allergic reaction.

AT WHAT AGE CAN ANAPHYLAXIS START?

Anaphylaxis can start at any age. There are no rules, except that it is more likely to occur in an atopic person – someone who has inherited the susceptibility to allergy.

WHAT ACTUALLY HAPPENS IN THE BODY?

When a susceptible person comes into contact with an allergen that causes an anaphylactic reaction to occur, that allergen becomes bound to the surface of the mast cells (see Chapter 1). The binding of the allergen to the surface of the mast cell causes it to release a number of different chemicals, or mediators, which have a profound effect on the organs of the body. In the skin they cause leakiness and relaxation of the small blood vessels, leading to flushing, swelling and characteristic rashes (urticaria and angio-oedema). In the lung they cause muscle spasm and narrowing of the airways, which become blocked and filled with mucus. In the gut there is also muscle spasm and leakiness of the blood vessels, causing colic and diarrhoea. The coronary arteries, which supply blood to the heart muscle, go into spasm, and damage to the muscle can occur. The veins collecting blood from the other organs of the body lose their tone and become larger and leaky, no longer doing their job properly. The blood pressure falls and the blood supply to all the major organs is compromised.

WHAT ARE THE SYMPTOMS?

The symptoms of anaphylaxis can vary in both severity and the speed with which they happen (speed of onset). Any of the following symptoms may occur:

- tingling of the lips or in the mouth,
- flushing of the skin or a generalised rash,
- swelling of the lips, mouth, face or throat, or hands and feet,
- nasal congestion,
- sweating and/or dizziness,
- difficulty in swallowing or speaking,
- abdominal cramps, nausea, vomiting and diarrhoea,
- wheezy chest,
- feeling of faintness and deep anxiety,
- weakness,
- collapse,
- loss of consciousness.

WHAT FACTORS INCREASE THE SEVERITY AND SPEED OF AN ALLERGIC REACTION?

Certain factors can increase the severity and speed of an allergic reaction. They are:

- alcohol,
- exercise,
- the amount of allergen ingested,
- stress.

WHAT IS THE TREATMENT?

Prompt treatment of anaphylaxis is essential and may be life-saving. The mainstay of treatment is an injection of adrenaline (also called epinephrine). It is a very safe drug, which must be given as early in a reaction as possible. If appropriate, an asthma-relieving inhaler can be given as well.

It is also helpful if oxygen is given once medical help is available.

Antihistamines

Antihistamine medication is often used as the first line of treatment for the relief of a mild to moderate allergic reaction. The symptoms are caused by the chemical histamine, which is produced during the end-stages of an allergic reaction. Antihistamines work by blocking the action of this chemical, which thus reduces the symptoms of redness, itching, mucosal swelling, excess secretions (e.g. runny nose) and allergic skin rashes.

You can buy certain antihistamines 'over the counter' (without a prescription), but there are many different types, so it is essential that you discuss with your pharmacist or your GP or allergy specialist the most appropriate choice for you. This is particularly important if you are taking any other medication. You should also get advice about when to take the antihistamine. Remember that, if the symptoms get worse, you *must* proceed to adrenaline (see below).

Side-effects of antihistamines

Modern antihistamines (e.g. astemizole, cetirizine, loratadine) have very few side-effects. Be aware, though, that some of the older antihistamines can make you feel drowsy and affect your ability to operate machinery and to drive. At present there is no legislation governing the use of medicines when undertaking these tasks, but it is your responsibility not to do so if you have symptoms or side-effects that could affect your judgement. (This is also the case for some other medications and alcohol.)

The Table below should help you choose an appropriate antihistamine.

Category	Antihistamine	Brand name
Unlikely to affect your ability to drive or to operate machinery	Acrivastine Fexofenadine Loratadine	Semprex; Benadryl Allergy Relief Telfast Clarityn; Clarityn Allergy
Could affect your ability to drive or to operate machinery	Cetirizine	Zirtec
Likely to affect your ability to drive or to operate machinery	Brompheniramine Chlorpheniramine Clemastine Mequitazine Triprolidine Ketotifen	Dimotane Piriton Aller-eze; Tavegil Primalan Pharmalgen Zaditen
So sedating that they are used as sedatives for children	Promethazine Trimeprazine (alimemazine)	Phenergan Vallergan

Other side-effects associated with the use of certain antihistamines
In 1990 and 1992 the Medicines Control Agency (part of the Department of Health) issued safety warnings that terfenadine and astemizole could, in certain circumstances, be associated with the development of abnormal heart rhythms. The effect is rare and was found only in people who exceeded the manufacturer's daily dose or were taking other drugs that interacted with the histamine. Nevertheless, terfenadine has been withdrawn from use.

Adrenaline

Adrenaline (epinephrine) in its natural form is a stress hormone that is produced in your body by the adrenal glands. Adrenaline causes the 'fight or flight' reaction, which prepares your body for any stressful activity by speeding up your heart and increasing the flow of blood to your muscles.

The medicine adrenaline is given by injection during a severe allergic reaction, in order to aid the reversal of the life-threatening symptoms that are associated with anaphylaxis.

How does adrenaline work?
In anaphylactic shock the blood vessels leak, the airways (bronchial) tissues swell and the blood pressure drops, causing choking and collapse. Adrenaline acts quickly to constrict blood vessels, to relax the muscles in the lungs to improve breathing, to stimulate the heartbeat and to reverse swelling around the face and lips.

The EpiPen and, more recently, the Anapen auto-injector are the most usual ways to inject it. They are available as a pre-loaded syringe with a spring-activated concealed needle, which automatically injects a predetermined dose of adrenaline when the device is pushed firmly against the thigh. In most cases the benefits of the adrenaline are felt within seconds, although large adults might need two doses of the EpiPen. Anyone who is at risk of having an anaphylactic reaction should always carry two adrenaline injector pens. This is because the duration of action is short – if it takes a long time to obtain medical attention, the effects might begin to wear off and a second dose will be needed.

EpiPen The EpiPen is suitable for adults and for children weighing over 30kg. It should be available from any chemist, with a prescription. The syringe contains 0.3mg adrenaline.

EpiPen Junior As a general guide, the EpiPen Junior is suitable for infants and children under 30kg as 0.15mg of adrenaline. For infants under 15kg your GP or allergy specialist will advise on the most appropriate form of adrenaline.

Anapen The adult dose is 0.3mg of adrenaline.

Min-I-Jet This is a pre-filled adrenaline syringe containing 0.5–1.0mg (1:1000 strength) available for use by children over 12 and adults. It has been superseded by the auto-injector, as it is rather cumbersome to operate in an emergency (because it has to be assembled).

If the Min-I-Jet has been prescribed for children, some of the adrenaline is expelled from the syringe to leave, as near as possible, the correct quantity in the syringe. The amount required is calculated from the child's body weight.

Adrenaline should be kept at room temperature, otherwise it may degrade. If the temperature exceeds 30∞C the Anapen should be kept in the refrigerator. The EpiPen should *not* be refrigerated. For suggestions on how to keep the adrenaline at room temperature when in a hot climate, see Chapter 16 ('Holidays and Travelling').

Medihaler-Epi This was an adrenaline aerosol, which was used in the same way as an asthma inhaler (a device by which medication is inhaled to treat the symptoms of asthma). It was withdrawn in 1997, and there is as yet no replacement but adrenaline inhalers not licensed for use in the UK can be prescribed on a 'named patient basis'.

Side-effects of adrenaline

The most common side (unwanted) effects of adrenaline are trembling, palpitations (an awareness of the heart beat), sweating, a fast heart beat, nausea, vomiting, dizziness and a feeling of anxiety or tension. These are the normal effects of adrenaline, which soon wear off. In fact, some people don't even notice them when adrenaline is administered in the recommended dose.

WHICH MEDICATION – AND WHEN?

When to take, or give, medication is understandably a cause of great concern. The most common question asked by people who have experienced moderate to severe allergic reactions is: 'At what stage of an allergic reaction should the prescribed antihistamine and adrenaline be taken?' There is, unfortunately, no way of knowing in advance how severe a reaction will be, but a good general guide is:

- For symptoms such as a rash, sneezing or an itchy throat, where there is no shortness of breath or feeling faint, initially take/give the antihistamines.
- If the reaction develops to include symptoms such as shortness of breath or feeling faint, adrenaline should be administered without delay.
- If the reaction includes breathing difficulties or feeling faint from the very beginning, miss out the antihistamines and give the adrenaline immediately.

If adrenaline is necessary, an ambulance should also be called immediately, because the beneficial effects of adrenaline are short-lived and further treatment may be necessary.

Two things can threaten life in anaphylaxis:

- Difficulty breathing, when the air passages become restricted – due either to swelling in the throat and upper airways or to narrowing of the small airways as in asthma.
- Circulatory collapse, leading to inadequate supplies of oxygen to the tissues of the body.

If treatment with adrenaline is not given until the reaction becomes this severe, it is less likely to be successful.

If you are in doubt whether the reaction has progressed enough to warrant the adrenaline, it is best to go ahead and use it. The risk of not having the adrenaline when it is needed far outweighs the risk of taking or giving the adrenaline unnecessarily, which is negligible.

TREATMENT WHEN TAKING OTHER MEDICATION

If you have some other medical condition such as high blood pressure or an abnormal heart rhythm, or are on certain other medication, you should seek specialist advice.

Beta-blockers (used by people with high blood pressure) make adrenaline relatively ineffective. Other treatments are available and these should be discussed with your GP or allergy specialist without delay.

Asthma
People with asthma are at greater risk of developing a severe or even potentially fatal anaphylactic reaction. Therefore, if you are in any doubt as to whether your symptoms of wheezing and breathlessness

are due to straightforward asthma or are part of a severe allergic reaction, you should administer adrenaline without delay.

Anaphylaxis mistaken

Anaphylaxis can be mistaken for conditions that have similar symptoms, such as hyperventilation, panic attacks, alcohol intoxication and low blood sugar (hypoglycaemia). This is an important reason for wearing some sort of medical identification jewellery that will tell others of your condition if you are unable to do so yourself (see Chapter 5, 'Your Anaphylaxis Contingency Plan').

Fatal anaphylaxis

Fatal anaphylaxis is rare but, owing to a lot of media coverage over the past few years, deaths due to food allergy seem to be more common than they are. The actual number is not known but fatalities from nut/peanut anaphylaxis are thought to be about 1 in 2,000 severe reactions for males and 1 in 1,000 severe reactions for females. It is therefore essential to keep this risk in perspective.

The fact that you are reading this book means you are trying to find out all you can about anaphylaxis, so that you understand it and know what to do if it does occur. You are more likely to ensure that you wear emergency identification and more likely to check food labels and methods of food preparation. All of this not only reduces the risks of a reaction occurring but also increases the likelihood of your receiving prompt and correct treatment if it is required.

The importance of information and understanding about anaphylaxis for people with an allergy and for their friends, relatives and guardians should not be underestimated.

Anaphylaxis at school

This subject is discussed in Chapter 6.

MANAGEMENT OF A SEVERE ATTACK

Have a written action plan in place and follow it.

Anyone who receives emergency adrenaline should be taken to the hospital accident and emergency (A&E) department immediately. Dial 999 and inform the controller that the person is suffering from anaphylaxis. If symptoms persist, or improve and then recur, a second dose of adrenaline may be required.

SPEEDING UP THE TREATMENT IN AN EMERGENCY

- Always wear medical identification.
- Have an action plan for treatment that is:
  – accessible,
  – easy to read,
  – easy to understand,
  – easy to implement,
  – up to date,
  – in the correct language if you are abroad (see Chapter 16, 'Holidays and Travelling').
- Carry at least two syringes of adrenaline at all times.
- Carry an antihistamine at all times.
- Be confident about when to take the antihistamine and when adrenaline is required.
- Tell others about your allergy and action plan for treatment.
- Have access to a mobile phone and charger at all times for emergency use.
- Ensure that an ambulance is called even if you have administered the adrenaline and feel better. The person calling the ambulance should always state that you are having an anaphylactic reaction, as this is a medical emergency where time is of the essence.
- Get more information if you are unsure of any of the above.

It is always important to seek emergency medical help even if adrenaline has been administered. The duration of action of an adrenaline injection may be as short as 10 minutes and, if symptoms recur, further treatment such as antihistamines and corticosteroids (steroids) might be needed. It will also be necessary for the person to be observed for a suitable period of time to make sure that recovery is complete.

Once in hospital other medication may be given, including oxygen, fluids, antihistamines and corticosteroids.

Even with adequate treatment with adrenaline, repeat attacks have been known to occur up to eight hours later. For this reason observation in an A&E department is recommended for eight hours following life-threatening anaphylaxis, and four hours for milder reactions.

What to expect in the A&E department

The precise treatment you receive when you reach hospital will be specific to the severity of the reaction and your symptoms. The Table opposite is meant purely as a general guide.

HOW CAN YOU PREVENT FURTHER REACTIONS?

The only way to prevent further attacks is to avoid the substance that caused it. If you are unsure about the cause, it is essential to seek advice from your GP who may refer you to an allergy clinic (see Chapters 2 and 3).

THE ANAPHYLAXIS CAMPAIGN

The Anaphylaxis Campaign is a charity that provides advice, information and support to susceptible people and their families about all aspects of anaphylaxis.

The Campaign also highlights anaphylaxis issues to the government bodies that make decisions on food policy. The aim of this is to improve food manufacturing, labelling and preparation practices to help reduce the risks to susceptible people of consuming a substance that may trigger an allergic reaction. It is advisable for all people who are at risk of anaphylaxis and their families to join the Anaphylaxis Campaign (address in Appendix 1).

THE PHARMACY AND THE 'LITTLE RED BOOK'

Increasingly we look to the pharmacist for help and guidance. The Code of Ethics of the Royal Pharmaceutical Society of Great Britain states that 'pharmacists must do everything reasonably possible to help a person in need of emergency medicines or treatment'. In 1999, a guide was written for community pharmacists to use as a reference. Called *Emergency First Aid: professional standards*, it outlines the most appropriate treatment of medical situations that are likely to arise. It gives guidance on the action to be taken in life-threatening situations – including anaphylaxis – when it is believed that a pharmacist would be justified in administering certain medicines.

Every pharmacy in the UK has a copy of this book, which is certainly reassuring if you have a severe allergic reaction in the High Street!

WHAT TO EXPECT IN THE A&E DEPARTMENT

Action	Reason
You are lain down	In case of fainting because of the drop in blood pressure during anaphylaxis
A small plastic tube (intravenous cannula) is immediately inserted into a vein, usually in your hand or arm, and a 'drip' set up	To gain access before the veins shut down, so that medication and fluid can be administered
Adrenaline from a syringe (not an auto-injector) is given via the cannula – if not already given, or a second dose if required	Because the action of adrenaline reverses the symptoms of anaphylaxis
An oxygen mask is placed on your face	To increase the level of oxygen in your blood; the level drops during anaphylaxis as a direct result of the drop in blood pressure
You are attached to a machine that monitors your blood pressure	To check that your blood pressure is returning to normal levels
You may be given hydrocortisone or other corticosteroids via the cannula	To reduce the swelling associated with anaphylaxis
Treatment continues as above until you are stable	To stabilise your blood pressure
You will be kept in A&E for observation: about 4 hours for a mild reaction, 8 hours for a severe reaction or overnight if required	In case a secondary reaction occurs that requires treatment, and for monitoring purposes
You may be given hydrocortisone tablets to take at home for 1 to 3 days	To prevent the likelihood of a delayed or secondary reaction
Letter written to your GP	To keep the GP informed and so that another adrenaline auto-injector can be prescribed if it has been used. For referral to an allergy clinic if required.

FREQUENTLY ASKED QUESTIONS

When and how should I carry my EpiPen?
It should be carried with you at all times – in a pocket or a handbag or in a protective case.

Where should I store my supply of EpiPen?
EpiPen should be kept at room temperature and not refrigerated. If it is exposed to extreme heat or sunlight, the adrenaline will turn brown. Check that the adrenaline is clear by looking through the viewing window of the auto-injector.

Where do I inject the adrenaline?
EpiPen should only be injected into the outer thigh, through clothing if necessary. Do not inject EpiPen anywhere else. (Trainer EpiPens are available for teaching the injection technique.)

Can I use a second EpiPen?
Usually one pen is sufficient, but if symptoms do not improve or they get worse, a second EpiPen may be administered five minutes after the first one.

Why is it important to seek medical attention immediately after using the EpiPen?
Further treatment and observation in hospital may be necessary because the symptoms of anaphylaxis might return.

How do I discard my adrenaline auto-injector after use?
Place the auto-injector back in the plastic case and give it to the emergency services, who will dispose of it safely.

What should I do with my out-of-date EpiPens?
When you go to collect your new EpiPens, give the out-of-date ones to the pharmacist, who will dispose of them safely.

5
Your Anaphylaxis Contingency Plan

By taking all the precautions discussed in this book, you should rarely, if ever, have a severe reaction. Nevertheless, you may accidentally eat or drink something that you would normally avoid, so you should always have a contingency plan just in case. Also included in this chapter are some more general information and helpful hints.

EMERGENCY PACK

The emergency pack described below contains information and medication that may be required if you have a serious allergic reaction. It is recommended that you have access to this pack *at all times*.

Information card
This contains essential information about you and how your next of kin (NOK) can be contacted in an emergency.

EMERGENCY MEDICAL INFORMATION

Name: Mrs A L Lergy
Address: 140 Adrenaline Close, London HE 1P
Tel: (H) 0123 456 789 (W) 0987 654 321
NOK: (Husband) Mr E C Zema
Tel: 0111 222 333 **Mobile:** 07988 777 666

Medical Information
Severe allergy to: Milk and dairy products
Eggs

IN THE CASE OF A SEVERE ALLERGIC REACTION, *I REQUIRE ADRENALINE*
I carry adrenaline for emergency use. Please administer this in an emergency and then dial **999** for an ambulance.

Identification (ID)

Special medical identification is especially useful if you are unable to communicate your needs (you may be unconscious, breathless or unable to speak clearly). With this identification your medical condition can be diagnosed and the correct treatment given. The faster the diagnosis is made, the sooner the life-saving adrenaline can be given. (ID is discussed in more detail later in this chapter.)

Two adrenaline auto-injectors

It is essential to carry two adrenaline auto-injectors (EpiPen or Anapen). This is because, if the first one does not relieve the symptoms after five minutes, a second dose is required.

Antihistamine

When the symptoms of a reaction start, you will not usually know if it will develop into full-blown anaphylaxis. For this reason it is useful to take an antihistamine (tablets or syrup), which is sometimes enough to stop the reaction developing any further.

Mobile phone

A mobile phone is optional but is useful to communicate quickly with those who may be able to help in an emergency. This includes alerting nearby friends/family and for calling an ambulance.

Action plan

ACTION PLAN FOR USE IN SEVERE ANAPHYLAXIS

1. Remove the EpiPen (adrenaline auto-injector) from the yellow tube.
2. Remove the grey safety cap.
3. Inject the adrenaline by pressing the EpiPen firmly against the thigh (instructions on the side of the EpiPen).
4. Call 999 for a paramedic ambulance, stating that it is for an anaphylactic reaction (severe allergy).
5. Give a second dose of adrenaline if the first one has not taken effect after 5 minutes.
6. When the ambulance arrives, make sure the paramedic is given your Emergency Pack, including the used EpiPen.

The information cards in this emergency pack can be written with help from your GP or allergy specialist.

It is essential that you make up an emergency pack such as the one outlined above, and that friends and family know of its existence. If you have an anaphylactic reaction, the pack will make it possible for the correct procedures to be undertaken before paramedics arrive and take over. Precious seconds will be saved in administering life-saving medication. In anaphylaxis *time is of the essence*.

GENERAL PREPARATION

Below is a list for you to check that you are prepared in the event that you have an anaphylactic reaction.

MY EMERGENCY CHECKLIST

☐ I have made up an emergency pack.

☐ I have checked the contents of my emergency pack with my GP or allergy specialist.

☐ I keep a check on the 'use by' date of my antihistamines and adrenaline auto-injectors to ensure that they are always in date.

☐ If I use the adrenaline auto-injector(s), I always order replacement(s) immediately.

☐ I do not expose my adrenaline auto-injectors to extremes of temperature.

☐ I keep my friends, family and colleagues informed about my allergy and the contents of my emergency pack.

☐ My friends, family and colleagues have a 'role-play' practice from time to time (about every three months) of the procedures to be taken in an emergency, using the EpiPen or Anapen Trainer.

☐ If I have a mobile phone, I always keep it charged and have an in-car charger in case the batteries run flat when I am in my car.

☐ I have a visible note about my severe allergy on the dashboard of my car.

☐ I carry with me identification that explains about my severe allergy.

If you are able to tick all the boxes in the checklist above, you can rest assured that you are doing all you can in preparation for an emergency – which, hopefully, will never happen.

IDENTIFICATION (ID)

Even with the best will in the world, accidents do happen. So it is essential that you are prepared for the possibility of an allergic reaction that, at its worst, could be fatal.

In a medical emergency it is not always possible to give details about your medical condition, so carrying identification is an easy way to inform members of the public and the medical profession about your allergy. This gives vital information about your condition, thereby assisting diagnosis and speeding up treatment so that critical seconds are not lost. The earlier the life-saving adrenaline is given, the greater the chance of a positive outcome.

Types of ID

Jewellery
Identity jewellery generally comes in the form of a necklace, bracelet or watch. These are available from four major sources:

Golden Key This is a mail order company providing an engraving service for SOS ID: bracelets, necklaces, key rings and badges.
Medic-Alert Foundation The Foundation has a selection of identification jewellery with an internationally recognised medical symbol, engraved with your medical condition and a phone number for the emergency services to call for all your details. There are Medic-Alert affiliates throughout the world. An initial fee is charged, plus an annual fee.
Medi-Tag This is similar to the Medic-Alert system. The jewellery available is similar, plus a watch.
SOS Talisman A necklace or bracelet with an internationally recognised medical symbol is unscrewed to access a 'concertina' of information inside. Details are filled in by the wearer.

ID jewellery can be expensive. If you are on a low income, you may be able to get financial help from a local charity. Contact the company that you are considering buying from and they will probably be able to offer further advice on this.

Identity cards

These come as a card or laminated card, and can be obtained from many self-help organisations, such as the British Allergy Foundation and the UCB Institute of Allergy. If you have to complete the details yourself, it may be useful to get help from your GP or allergy specialist to ensure that the details and terminology are correct. (The ID cards on which you write your own details are available free of charge from the UCB Institute of Allergy.)

Badges

Some parents make or have made material, metal or plastic badges that announce their child's allergy such as 'Do not give me nuts' or 'I am allergic to eggs'. This can make some children feel special but others may feel the odd one out. Nevertheless, it is important to keep people informed about a child's allergy without making the child feel isolated or 'different'. (Contact Davies Engraving or AAIA for children's badges – addresses in Appendix 1.)

Tags

Local key cutters and engravers will often make up key rings or tags (or anything else you can suggest) with ID details. Some people find that this method of identification suits their needs.

Helpful hints

- If you have to fill in any medical details on the ID, ask your GP or allergy specialist to help you, or to check what you have written.
- ID should be carried at all times.
- ID should be visible.
- The information provided on the ID should be correct and up to date.
- If you are travelling to a foreign country, the ID should be modified or alternative information provided so that the people there can understand it (see Chapter 16, 'Holidays and Travelling').
- If your ID carries a yearly fee, make sure that this is paid (perhaps by Direct Debit), so that your details remain on the database. Failure to pay could render your ID invalid.

6
Anaphylaxis
and Going to School

Anaphylaxis is relatively rare, whereas food allergy causing very unpleasant but not life-threatening symptoms is common. Bear in mind, too, that the severity of allergic reactions can change over time – some children's decreasing but some increasing. This chapter deals with the serious, possibly life-threatening, allergic reaction that might affect your child when at school.

PRE-SCHOOL

Pre-school children are usually too young to know how to avoid foods to which they are allergic. Food is usually a large part of their day, which is broken up by snack and meal breaks. As the child's parents, you play a key role in this situation. It is your responsibility to make sure that there are suitable snacks and treats available for everyday activities and special activities. You should liase closely with the class teacher and the parents of the other children. As always, it is essential to have an action plan for emergency use, which should be reviewed regularly.

MEDICAL QUESTIONNAIRE

Parents are usually required to complete a medical questionnaire when their child joins a new school. Some schools now include questions that are designed to identify children with allergies to foods, latex and venom.

A child at risk of anaphylaxis presents a challenge to any school. However, with the correct plans, information and co-ordination, school life can continue as normal. Each child should have an action plan devised for use in an emergency.

SETTING UP AN ACTION PLAN

For a child who has a severe food allergy, the parents, teachers and others will make considerable efforts to try to ensure that as many risks as possible are reduced. Useful leaflets about anaphylaxis at school include *Anaphylaxis and Schools: how we can make it work* (Anaphylaxis Campaign) and *Information for Parents and Schools – anaphylaxis: child-specific protocol* (British Allergy Foundation). However, with the best will in the world, accidents can still happen. If they do, it is essential that everyone around at the time knows what to expect and what is expected of them.

Child-specific action plan

Sample child-specific action plans (or protocols) are available from the British Allergy Foundation and the Anaphylaxis Campaign. They have a standard format and will help you to complete a plan that is specific to your child. The best way to achieve this is to formulate a plan in association with the school nurse, the nursery/school staff, the head teacher, the allergy specialist, the GP, the school health and safety co-ordinator and the local education authority. The final version should then be distributed to everyone concerned.

The plan deals with all of the important issues, including:

- Anaphylaxis – what it is, and why a protocol is required to ensure the child's safety.
- Identification – ensuring that the child is known to be at risk.
- Consent and agreement – between the parents or guardians and the school.
- Emergency procedure – the action to take, including guidance on administering adrenaline and obtaining medical help (dialling 999).
- Food management – how to prevent reactions.
- Medication – antihistamines, adrenaline.
- Professional indemnity – for school staff willing to give emergency treatment.
- Reducing the risks – the emergency/action plan, having role-play periodically (e.g. every term).
- Staff training – relevant literature and videos about the allergy, having role-play, training in administering the medication.
- What to tell the other children.

The plan is in place not only for your child's safety but also to help the school staff, and will bring with it security and assurance. It is helpful if the plan is role-played so as to aid speed and understanding in the event of an anaphylactic reaction.

Action For Anaphylaxis is a video available from the Anaphylaxis Campaign. It is about a child having an anaphylactic reaction at school and how it was managed successfully – using an action plan. It would be useful for the school to obtain a copy of this for training purposes. Bring it to the attention of the school staff when you are formulating the action plan, as they may be unaware of its existence. Tell them also about the literature that is available from the Anaphylaxis Campaign, which they might find useful.

The Department for Education and Employment and the Department of Health have jointly produced a pack for schools, called *Supporting Pupils with Medical Needs*. Its purpose is to help schools draw up policies on managing medication. It includes a section on anaphylaxis and its management.

Sample action plan (protocol)
The action plan below is based on the protocol by the Anaphylaxis Campaign, which was compiled from working documents in use for children in schools in Birmingham, Dudley, Berkshire and Hampshire. (The schools and local education authorities have kindly shared them with the Anaphylaxis Campaign.) This action plan is for guidance only. The one for your child should be developed according to the GP's or the consultant's judgement.

---

1 Background

1.1 It is thought that John could have an anaphylactic reaction if he eats nuts or products containing nuts.
If this happens, he is likely to need medical attention; in an extreme situation, his condition may be life-threatening. However, medical advice is that attention to his diet – in particular the exclusion of nuts – together with the availability of his emergency medication, are all that is necessary. In all other respects, his doctor recommends that his education should carry on 'as normal'.

1.2 John also has a mild asthmatic condition, and may therefore need occasional access to his inhaler.

1.3   The arrangements set out below are intended to help John, his parents and the school in achieving the least possible disruption to his education but also to make appropriate provision for his medical requirements.

2   Details

2.1   The head teacher will arrange for the teachers and other staff in the school to be briefed about John's condition and about the arrangements listed in this document.

2.2   John's parents will provide for him:
   • a suitable mid-morning snack
   • a suitable packed lunch
   • suitable sweets to be considered as treats, and to be kept by the class teacher.

2.3   The school staff will take all reasonable steps to ensure that John does not eat any food items unless they have been prepared or approved by his parents.

2.4   John's parents will remind him regularly of the need to refuse any food items that might be offered to him by other pupils.

2.5   If there are any proposals that mean John might leave the school site, discussions will be held first between the school and John's parents in order to agree appropriate provision and safe handling of his medication.

2.6   Whenever the planned curriculum involves cookery or experimentation with food items, discussion will be held first between the school and John's parents to agree procedures and suitable alternatives.

2.7   The school will hold, under secure conditions, appropriate medication, clearly marked for use by designated school staff or qualified personnel, and showing an expiry date.

2.8   A bottle of loratadine medicine and two EpiPens are to be held in the head teacher's office. John's parents accept responsibility for supplying and maintaining appropriate up-to-date medication.

3   Allergic reaction

3.1   If John shows any physical symptoms for which there is no obvious alternative explanation, his condition will be reported immediately to the head teacher or teacher in charge. On receiving such a report, the person in charge, if agreeing that John's condition gives cause for concern, will instruct a staff member to contact, in direct order of priority: *cont.*

- Ambulance/Emergency services 999
- GP 0447 5894/0447 6894
- local health centre: 0447 8891
  with the message: **John Smith, an anaphylactic reaction**
  and then, in the following order:
- mother: 0447 6651
- father: 0343 6752
- grandparents: 0656 7878
- Mrs Jones (neighbour) 0447 4345

3.2   While waiting for medical assistance, the head teacher and designated staff will assess John's condition and administer the appropriate medication in line with the perceived symptoms and following closely the instructions given by the doctor during the staff training session.

3.3   The procedure given below will be followed:

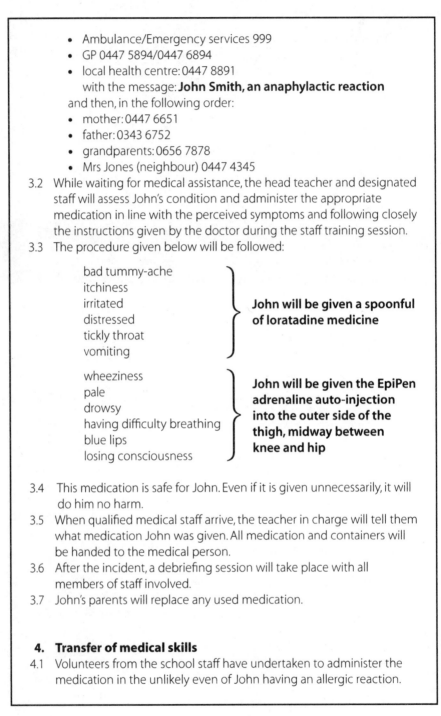

bad tummy-ache
itchiness
irritated
distressed
tickly throat
vomiting

John will be given a spoonful of loratadine medicine

wheeziness
pale
drowsy
having difficulty breathing
blue lips
losing consciousness

John will be given the EpiPen adrenaline auto-injection into the outer side of the thigh, midway between knee and hip

3.4   This medication is safe for John. Even if it is given unnecessarily, it will do him no harm.

3.5   When qualified medical staff arrive, the teacher in charge will tell them what medication John was given. All medication and containers will be handed to the medical person.

3.6   After the incident, a debriefing session will take place with all members of staff involved.

3.7   John's parents will replace any used medication.

4.   Transfer of medical skills

4.1   Volunteers from the school staff have undertaken to administer the medication in the unlikely even of John having an allergic reaction.

4.2   A training session was attended by seven members of the school staff. Dr T Fox, the community paediatrician, explained in detail John's condition, the symptoms of the anaphylactic reaction, and the stages and procedures for the administration of medication.

4.3   Advice is available to the school staff at any point in the future when they feel the need for further assistance. The medical training will be repeated at the beginning of the next academic year.

4.4   The local authority indemnifies any member of the school staff who agrees to administer medication to John in school, given the full agreement of his parents and the school.

Staff indemnity

The local authority fully indemnifies its staff against claims for alleged negligence, provided they are acting within the scope of their employment, have been provided with adequate training and are following the local education authority's guidelines. For the purposes of indemnity, the administration of medicines falls within this definition and hence the staff can be reassured about the protection their employer provides. The indemnity covers the consequences that might arise when an incorrect dose is given inadvertently or where the medication is not given. In practice, indemnity means that the local authority, not the employee, would meet the cost of damages, if a claim for alleged negligence were successful. It is very rare for school staff to be sued for negligence; the action is usually between the parent and the employer.

5.   Agreement and conclusion

5.1   A copy of these notes will be held by the school and by the parents. A copy will be sent to Dr Fox, the GP and the local education authority, for information.

5.2   Any revisions necessary will be the subject of further discussion between the school and the parents.

5.3   Any changes in routine will be noted and circulated on a termly basis.

Agreed and signed by

Head teacher _____ Date _____

Chair of Governing Body _____ Date _____

Parents of John Smith _____ Date _____

Copies of the action plan should be held by the school, the parents, the GP and the local education authority. It is essential that all parties be kept informed of any changes and agree any amendments. The action plan should have the date clearly marked so that old versions can be discarded and do not get mixed up with the updates.

Summary of action to take for a severe reaction

Action	Reason
Delegate someone to call 999 for an ambulance, stating that the child is having an anaphylactic reaction	So you may stay with and reassure the child
Lie the child down on his or her side, immediately	To minimise the drop in blood pressure that is characteristic of an anaphylactic reaction (the child might faint)
Give adrenaline when breathing is laboured or the child is floppy or unconscious	To reverse the symptoms of anaphylaxis
Delegate someone to call the parents (do not leave the child alone)	To keep parents informed and so they come to provide support for the child as soon as possible
On arrival of the ambulance: parent (or staff member if the parent is not there) to go with the ambulance to nearest A&E department	Support for the child and to provide information about the child and the reaction/treatment given

HEALTH AND SAFETY IN SCHOOL

It is the duty of school staff to safeguard the health of pupils. Although teachers have a general legal duty to act on behalf of the parents (*in loco parentis*) they are *not* responsible for administering or supervising pupils taking medication. Some staff may, however, volunteer to undertake appropriate training to enable them to do so.

All schools are required to have a policy for calling an ambulance if it is required. Treatment will usually begin when the ambulance staff arrive; this is appropriate for most incidents. There are, however, certain conditions that require immediate treatment and cannot wait for the ambulance. One such condition is anaphylaxis.

Medical training of school staff
This is usually done by the GP, school doctor or paediatrician, and sometimes by the community paediatric nurse, health visitor or school nurse. Teachers will have the opportunity to practise giving the injections and to have their questions answered. The agreed action plan may also be discussed. Certificates of competence are sometimes given. There are no formal nationally agreed standards, so training will vary.

If this training has not been carried out in your child's school, ask your GP to contact the school nurse, who will arrange for it to be done.

Issues for the school staff
Indemnity for school staff is an important issue, and the lack of it has, in the past, discouraged many from volunteering to administer medication. The teachers' unions advise their members that, if they agree to take on this responsibility, they should follow strictly controlled guidelines and obtain professional indemnity from their employers, to cover them in cases of alleged negligence.

The school or the local education authority often provides indemnity as a matter of course. It is the responsibility of individual school staff members to ensure they are fully covered for action they might take within the scope of their employment.

Medication at school
Schools have their own policy on the storage of medication. They may allow pupils to carry it or it may be held by the class teacher or in the secretaries' office. On no account should it be kept in a locked cupboard, because there might be a delay in getting it if the keys cannot be located. It would be wise for you to check the school's policy and, if necessary, negotiate a suitable compromise.

Some schools have a policy of locking away all medication. The main reasons for this are worries that the child will lose the medication or that it will be misused by another child. If your child's school has such a policy, discuss it with the head teacher. It may also be worth getting the GP to write to the head teacher with his or her recommendations regarding your child carrying the medication or where and how medication should be stored at school.

RECORDS

It is essential that a record be kept of any allergic reaction that occurs. The information should be dated and signed by the staff involved in the treatment. Details of mild and more severe reactions and their causes, location, etc., can be useful in preventing future reactions. For example, if every reaction happens at lunch time despite your child taking a packed lunch from home, it could indicate that sandwiches are being swapped, with the result that your child sometimes eats peanut butter, which is a trigger food.

FOOD AT SCHOOL

It is understandable that you may be concerned about your child eating in a place where there are many potentially harmful foods around. However, eating with friends is an important part of fitting in and social integration.

Although some parents prefer to provide all their child's food for consumption at school, others are happy to trust the school caterers to provide suitable food. It is sensible, though, to formulate a code of practice that will encompass a particular child's special dietary needs and ensure that only correct food is provided. The Anaphylaxis Campaign can help with this.

To handle the growing problem of pupils with food allergy, some schools create a peanut/nut-free or milk-free table for children to eat at. They also establish a no-food-trading policy, as children swapping food with each other is a major reason for allergic reactions at school.

Make sure that your child knows what foods cause an allergic reaction and the importance of avoiding them. Role-play possible scenarios to help your child feel confident when dealing with situations relating to eating and the allergy – for example, peer pressure, teasing, bullying or just ordinary temptation to eat an offending food.

Sometimes the will to protect children physically can result in harming them psychologically. So it is difficult – but important – to get the balance right. There are many ways of keeping others informed about your child's allergy, including:

- educating your child not to accept food from others,
- joining an allergy support group,

- talking to people, explaining about the allergy,
- using the Anaphylaxis Campaign literature and videos.

Before your child attends a new school, schedule a meeting with the teachers, school nurse, catering staff and office staff. Explain to them about the allergy, which foods cause a reaction and precautions that must be taken. They should also be told about the emergency procedure that should be followed (the action plan), reading food labels and lunch time considerations such as:

- who sits with whom, and with which food,
- going home for lunch,
- your attending at lunchtime to supervise,
- whether your child should eat food provided by the school or bring food from home.

Banning foods from the school

Banning a particular food is one option in a school's management of food allergies. Doing this can, however, have associated problems:

- It creates a false sense of security, because pupils feel confident to eat any foods that are offered to them at school, when staff do not realise that it is not just peanut butter and Snickers that contain nut/peanut derivatives.
- Some parents might see this as an imposition, especially if it is going to be disadvantageous to their child. For example, nuts/peanuts are an important source of protein for vegetarians or vegans, or an underweight fussy child will eat only peanut butter sandwiches. Bans are likely to leave parents feeling cross rather than creating a harmonious, safe environment for the allergic child.
- For a ban to work effectively, everyone involved would have to constantly read food labels and call manufacturers to determine whether their food products contain the trigger food. This would be unrealistic.
- If all parents of children with severe food allergies requested that the offending foods be removed from the school, the resulting diet would become very limited and everyone would be confused as well as irate!
- Creating a ban would be likely to stigmatise the allergic child.

- Banning a food from the school creates a false situation and does not teach the child how to live with the allergy. When they eventually leave school they will be unprepared for life in the real world.

SCHOOL ACTIVITIES

Review plans for any activities that may involve food (e.g. parties, trips, cooking, crafts) on a monthly or half-term basis so that plans can be made to allow your child to participate in them safely. If your child is to go on a school trip, make sure that everyone involved in providing refreshments on the outing is given plenty of notice about suitable food and drink.

Unsuitable activities

Certain class activities – for example, cookery classes, craft lessons, custard pie competition – may be unsafe. It is important that children who cannot take part in these activities are given related alternative tasks. Otherwise, both they and their fellow pupils might feel alienated. Work with the school staff to find a suitable solution to this sort of problem.

7
Anaphylaxis in Young Adults

It is a fact that anaphylaxis can be fatal, although this is very rare. In recent years the victims have tended to be young people in their late teens or early twenties. Perhaps this is partly because people in this age group tend to take more risks or are more susceptible to peer pressure to 'fit in'. Whatever the reason, it has become tragically apparent that some lives could have been saved if the victims had had a greater understanding of their condition, had carried adrenaline with them and had taken more care in selecting food when eating away from home.

Recognising these facts, in 1999 the Anaphylaxis Campaign distributed thousands of information booklets to students throughout the UK. The booklet gave the following tips to help people with a severe allergy to live a normal and full life:

- Face up to your allergy – don't ignore it, hoping it will go away.
- Read food labels. It takes only seconds and could save your life.
- When eating out, be direct with waiters and catering staff.
- Avoid eating in high-risk places: for example, the food in Indian and Oriental restaurants often has nuts and peanuts among the ingredients, and misunderstandings can occur among staff who don't speak much English.
- Don't handle this alone – educate your friends about your allergy.
- Be alert to all symptoms. Don't ignore them.
- If you have an adrenaline kit, make sure you take it everywhere.

The Anaphylaxis Campaign runs workshops and education groups designed to help young people who are at risk of anaphylaxis to understand and manage their allergy and to develop confidence. The information should help them in the everyday situations that can put them at risk as well as knowing how to avoid needless restrictions. This knowledge should reduce the incidence of both anaphylaxis and fatalities: if a reaction does occur, the adrenaline will be readily available and administered correctly.

COLLEGE STUDENTS LIVING-IN

If you are a college or university student, you should inform staff, room mates and hall mates about the foods that cause an allergic reaction, symptoms to be aware of and action to take if a reaction occurs.

Keep your medication in an easily accessible place, and a laminated up-to-date action plan by the phone.

EXTRA TIPS

- Too much alcohol can affect your judgement and speed up an allergic reaction, so beware!
- Before you kiss, check what your partner has been eating; it may be unsafe to do so until they have washed and cleaned their teeth.
- Exercise can speed up the rate of a reaction; slow down if you suspect a reaction may be coming on.
- A food to which you are allergic can turn up unexpectedly, so always check food ingredient labels. If there is no label, don't eat the food but find something that is definitely safe for you to eat.
- Put yourself in your friends' position. Would you find it a problem if they told you they have to be careful about what they eat and have to carry medication around just in case they eat something they shouldn't? And, by the way, could you learn how to administer it just in case they are too ill? Would you mind? Of course not! In fact, you would probably feel quite pleased that you were trusted to do this.

If you want more information, try the various websites listed in Appendix 2. Some websites have pages dedicated to teenagers and young adults.

Enjoying Food

8
The Dietitian's Role

If you wish to see a dietitian for dietary advice, you need a referral from either your GP or a hospital consultant. Any hospital consultant and many GPs can refer a patient to the dietitian but it is usually by a dermatologist, chest physician or allergy specialist because they are the specialists who see the people with allergies.

GETTING A REFERRAL

Even if you decide to see a dietitian privately, you still need a referral. This is to protect you from dietary advice that might adversely affect an ongoing medical condition or treatment. After your appointment, it is usual for the dietitian to send a letter to the referring doctor to inform them of the nutritional advice you have been given. The doctor then files this information in your medical notes for future reference.

Unfortunately, some people choose to see a 'nutritionist', 'nutritional therapist' or similar person who may have only very limited or no medical qualifications. In addition, they are not state registered and are therefore not bound by any national regulations. You do not need a doctor's referral to see them, and their treatment may be damaging if they do not know your full medical history. The other drawback is that follow-up care may not be given after you are placed on a restricted diet, which is dangerous. The following scenario is more common than is often realised.

Julie has had allergy testing and has been told to avoid all dairy products, wheat, red meat, citrus fruits and soya. Without expert follow-up care she has remained on a restricted diet for some time, believing that it is good for her health. It is only when Julie begins to feel unwell and goes to her GP for advice that she is referred to a dietitian for 'unexplained weight loss and anaemia' and she is diagnosed with malnutrition.

Such potentially harmful consequences can occur because:

- the poorly qualified/unqualified 'therapist' has a poor knowledge and understanding of the possible nutritional implications of placing someone on a restricted diet and not giving them follow-up care for prolonged periods of time,
- the individual has a poor understanding of the prescribed diet and may not realise that new symptoms are related to it,
- the individual cannot afford to go back and see the 'therapist' for on-going care.

This is why it is essential to see a fully qualified dietitian.

SEEING THE DIETITIAN

When you go to see the dietitian, it will be useful if you are prepared and know what to expect so that you can get the most from your visit.

The allergen is known

If you have had a severe allergic reaction to food and the allergen causing it was easily identifiable, the dietitian will advise you about completely excluding that food and its derivatives from your diet, and will suggest replacement foods to maintain good health.

The allergen is not known

If you have had a severe allergic reaction but the cause was unknown, you will have been referred for allergy testing (see Chapters 2 and 3) before you see the dietitian. Once the likely cause of the allergy has been identified, the dietitian will advise you on how to avoid the culprit and its derivatives whilst maintaining a balanced diet.

If your reaction was not a severe one, elimination of suspect food(s) for a specific length of time followed by a 'food challenge' may be useful. Three dietary approaches are commonly used: exclusion, elimination and few foods.

Exclusion diet

This involves excluding one or two foods that are suspected of causing a reaction. The diet is usually followed for two to four weeks to assess any changes in your symptoms. During this period it is essential that you keep an accurate food and symptom diary. The foods are then re-introduced, while you continue keeping the diary. From your response(s), it is then possible for the dietitian to give you advice on which foods to avoid and which to continue to eat.

Date	Time	Food/Drink consumed	Time	Symptoms

Figure 8.1 Example of a food and symptom diary

Elimination diet

This starts with a full diet and then taking foods from the diet, one by one, keeping a food and symptom diary all the time. The most common allergens and suspect foods are removed from the diet first. Once the reactions have stopped or improved, the foods are reintroduced to the diet, one by one, all the time noting any reactions. This process can take months but, with skin-prick and RAST tests, usually leads to a completely accurate diagnosis. To achieve this, though, it is essential that you keep an accurate diary.

Few foods diet

This diet consists of a small number of basic foods (e.g. lamb, pears, sugar, rice, water), the aim being to exclude all major food allergens. This is followed for up to two weeks. If you improve, the omitted foods are systematically reintroduced into your diet every few days to identify the offending food.

If there has been no improvement after the initial two weeks, the few foods left in the diet may be removed and you will be placed on a special formula drink for a few days. This will show if the food causing the reaction was one of the 'few foods'. It is very rare to have to go to such drastic measures, as the initial few foods diet is usually enough to get rid of the symptoms.

For advice on which foods to avoid for specific diets, see Chapter 10 ('Special Diets'). Remember, though, that the information given there is meant as a guide only and following any such diets *must* be done under the strict supervision of a dietitian.

Factors to discuss with your dietitian

When you are going to embark on a special diet, discuss with your dietitian:

- the aim of the diet, to make sure you understand it and how to follow it,
- what is the likely cost of the foods (they can be considerably more expensive than 'ordinary' food),
- making sure that your diet is nutritious,
- how long you will be on the diet,
- how to manage when eating out, including holidays, business travel, work lunches, celebrations and social events,
- what treats you are allowed,
- your general health,
- any medication that you are taking (e.g. antihistamines) and whether you carry adrenaline with you at all times,
- how often you should contact the dietitian,
- how much support the dietitian will be able to give you and when,
- withdrawal symptoms (e.g. headache, lethargy) in the first few days of the diet.

The dietitian will be able to advise you or give you information about many aspects. The list below is in alphabetical order, and the importance of the entries will be specific to your particular needs. Some of them will be more relevant if you are following a diet involving the long-term avoidance of a particular food. For example:

- adapting existing recipes,
- baby formulas,
- comprehensive list of foods to avoid,
- contact by phone in case of queries,
- cookbooks, new recipes and cooking tips,
- eating away from home/celebrations,
- encouragement and support,
- Food Intolerance Databank,
- food manufacturers' information and 'free from' lists,
- ideas to help add variety and palatability to your diet,
- information on food labelling to aid understanding and interpretation,
- long-term guidance on avoidance if required, including support groups,
- nutrient supplementation,
- nutritional adequacy of your diet, diet sheets and meal plans,
- products available on prescription,

- replacement or substitute foods,
- review appointments,
- supermarket 'free from' lists,
- translations of food information, for travelling abroad,
- written advice as required.

Problems may arise either during the restricted diet or in the reintro-duction phase. For example, sometimes the diet isn't fully understood and isn't followed properly, which can give false positive or false nega-tive results. Parents can sometimes become obsessed with their child's special diet, risking the possibility of the child rebelling and eating 'banned' food secretly. Occasionally, people restrict their diet in other ways that they are reluctant to tell the dietitian – who then is unaware of their risk of nutritional deficiency. Also, if you follow the prescribed diet for too long and don't see the dietitian for check-ups and advice, you could suffer from malnutrition. People sometimes feel that, because they are doing well on the restricted diet, they don't want to risk reintroducing foods in case the symptoms return. If you are taking medication (e.g. antihistamines) or having complementary therapies such as acupuncture or homoeopathy or even undergoing changes in your lifestyle, these may mask the effects of foods being reintroduced into your diet, resulting in false or inconclusive results.

Factors that you need to consider when following a restricted diet include:

- being organised about food shopping and cooking,
- shopping: location and opening hours of specialist shops, and which substitute foods to buy,
- having confidence to explain your needs,
- your cooking skills,
- the cost,
- your feelings of deprivation,
- social isolation,
- whether meals should be kept separate or all the family to eat the same food,
- nutrition,
- taste: acceptability of substitute foods, bland diet, etc.

The pitfalls of following a restricted diet include:

- you cannot afford the diet,
- you are already avoiding other foods (e.g. you are a vegan or

vegetarian, your food preferences, food intolerances, your culture),
- not following the diet properly under qualified supervision,
- your cooking skills are poor,
- parents feel guilty,
- you don't really understand the diet,
- you don't keep strictly to the diet (poor compliance),
- you are given conflicting advice.

In general, you are more likely to follow the diet successfully if you understand the diet and the reason for it, and are well motivated, with the necessary resources, time and money.

It is only worth embarking on a restricted diet if you are prepared to adhere completely to the diet and to keep a precise food and symptom diary. This will not be easy but your perseverance will usually be rewarded by being able to identify the foods that are causing the discomfort.

If the symptoms are only mild, you may decide that the diet restrictions are worse than the symptoms! Long-term adherence to a diet is recommended only if there is definite proof of the benefits.

It is not ideal to commence a restricted diet if you:

- are reluctant to do it,
- are malnourished or underweight,
- are depressed,
- are in a sports training programme for competition,
- are a pregnant woman or are breast-feeding,
- have food-related psychiatric disorder (e.g. anorexia nervosa or bulimia),
- have an illness in which fatigue is a major symptom (e.g. post-viral syndrome/ME),
- have a disease (e.g. Crohn's disease) that can affect your nutritional status – for example, one that affects appetite, digestion, metabolism or absorption of nutrients, or causes nausea or vomiting,
- have major celebration or holiday looming.

Before you embark on the diet, it is important to discuss fully any such issues with your specialist.

OTHER INFORMATION THAT MAY BE REQUIRED BY THE DIETITIAN

The dietitian is likely to ask you to keep a diet diary, to record the pattern of your meals, the type of food you eat and fluids you drink, your method(s) of cooking, how many meals and snacks you have a day and what they contain, and how often you miss a meal. You will also usually be asked to keep a note of any symptoms you have while following the diet. It will be useful for the dietitian to have information about:

- other diets you have tried and their outcome,
- any known or suspected intolerances or allergies,
- your food likes, dislikes and cravings,
- your willingness to try substitute foods.

Also pertinent will be information about home cooking facilities, who prepares the meals and who does the shopping.

9
Food Labelling

This chapter discusses current food-labelling laws and initiatives by the food industry that will help you to identify and choose suitable products for your special diet.

If you are allergic or intolerant to a food, it is relatively easy to avoid it in its natural state. However, avoiding derivatives of that food in manufactured products, when it is a 'hidden' ingredient, is somewhat trickier. It is therefore essential for you to know exactly what you are trying to avoid and look for it on the food ingredients label.

By law, food labels must list all the ingredients, in order of weight. This list can get very lengthy and sometimes quite confusing – especially when a product contains many chemicals and E-numbers. Don't be put off by this. As long as you are sure what you are looking for on a label, you can make the right food choices.

PRODUCT CHANGES

Manufacturers sometimes change the formulation of their products. This may happen when a supplier changes, or with recipe developments. A previously safe food can then become unsafe. Because of this, it is essential that you check labels *every* time you purchase a food. Never get complacent and assume a food is safe to eat because you have had it before.

CURRENT FOOD-LABELLING LAW

In 1991 the Government published the Green Paper about food labelling regulations. It stressed the need for universal labelling guidelines. The result was the Food Labelling Regulations 1996, specifying the labelling for pre-packed foods for Great Britain. These Regulations were modified in February 2000.

Current food-labelling law states that food packaging must give:

- the name of the food,
- a list of the key ingredients, in descending order of the quantities it contains (but see the note, below),
- a 'use by' or 'best before' date,
- any special storage and/or cooking instructions,
- the name and address of the manufacturer or packager,
- information on the process used in manufacture (e.g. dried, frozen, smoked),
- the presence of genetically modified (GM) or irradiated ingredients.

Notes

1. Ingredients do not have to be listed if they are part of another, compound, ingredient that makes up less than 25% of the final product (see 'The 25% rule' below).
2. Some ingredients, such as some flavourings and additives, do not have to be listed.

THE '25% RULE'

Because of the 25% exemption (in Note 1, above) applying to compound ingredients, the presence of small amounts of an allergen may legally be undeclared on pre-packaged foods. Since 1993 the EU has been discussing an amendment under which nuts, peanuts, eggs, cow's milk, fish, shellfish, soya and sesame seeds would be excluded from this rule. They would all have to be clearly labelled whether a compound ingredient or not.

Following recent discussions by the Codex Alimentarius (see below), this issue should soon be resolved – which will be welcome news for everyone with a food allergy. Until this happens we can be grateful that many food manufacturers and retailers produce 'free from' lists and clear allergen labelling on their products, which makes it easier to identify products that are suitable for special diets.

Codex Alimentarius

Codex Alimentarius is a system of international food standards, sponsored by the United Nations and based with its Food and Agriculture Organization (FAO) in Rome. Over 160 member states are represented on it. Although not legally binding, its standards are generally respected and influence both individual governments and bodies such as the EU. There is still debate about whether the 25% rule should be dropped when dealing with potential food allergens.

HELP! THERE ARE NO INGREDIENTS LISTED

Some foods sold in the catering sector or at in-store service counters don't have to carry an ingredients list. These are:

- fresh fruit and vegetables that have not been peeled or cut up,
- plain carbonated water,
- vinegar,
- cheese, butter and fermented milk or cream with no additional ingredients,
- flour fortified in accordance with the bread and flour regulations,
- drinks with an alcohol content of more than 1.2% by volume,
- single-ingredient foods.

These foods are exempt from labelling requirements because of the condition in which they are sold. Food that is not pre-packaged or which has been pre-packed for direct sale (e.g. that sold in bakeries, delicatessens and butchers) need only indicate its name, the presence of certain types of additives, and the presence of ingredients that have been irradiated or derived from genetically modified soya or maize.

There may be an in-store product guide that holds information on the ingredients of these unlabelled products, so ask for assistance from the vendor. If you are unsure about the ingredients of a product, do not under any circumstances eat it if there is a chance that it may contain an ingredient to which you are allergic. If you do, the consequences might be serious.

Ingredients not mentioned in the ingredients list

The following foods don't have to be mentioned on the ingredients list:

- Additives used as processing aids (e.g. antioxidant, modified starch).
- Substances used as solvents or as 'carriers' for additives.
- Additives 'carried over' into a food by one of its ingredients if they serve no significant technological function in the final food.

- Constituents of ingredients temporarily separated during manufacture which are later reintroduced in their original proportions.

'MAY CONTAIN'

An increasing number of food manufacturers are adding to their packaging the declaration 'This product may contain traces of nuts/peanuts' (or other allergenic ingredients). The aim is to highlight products that might have been in contact with that allergen – for example, by being baked in a contaminated tin or by passing along a contaminated production line (see also Chapter 15, 'Cross-contamination'). In some instances, such a label may be put on a product even if the chance of cross-contamination is minuscule. This has resulted in many products that do not contain nuts/peanuts, and were previously suitable for someone allergic to nuts/peanuts, now becoming out of bounds. The public's response to this practice has not been favourable, because it has reduced the food choices available to anyone with that food allergy. Some people are therefore now unnecessarily avoiding foods that were previously regarded as – and may still be – safe.

On the other hand, many people – especially teenagers – ignore 'may contain' warnings, believing that the warnings are a cop-out and don't represent a real risk. This is not sensible, and you should always heed such labels. They now enable people to identify a reason for previously unknown allergic reactions, and they can avoid the suspect food or ingredient.

The Institute of Grocer Distribution, which includes a representative from the Anaphylaxis Campaign, has drawn up a Code of Practice for the labelling of serious allergens. In an effort to reduce the need to use the 'may contain' warning, they stress the importance of good manufacturing practice, which should eliminate accidental inclusion of allergens. They also stress the need for improved education and awareness of food allergy issues in food retail outlets and restaurants.

THE FOOD INDUSTRY'S RESPONSE TO THE FOOD ALLERGY PROBLEM

Several widely publicised deaths linked to food allergies (nut/peanut allergies in particular) have increased awareness among the public, the food industry and the medical profession. Since the early 1990s many initiatives have been developed to reduce the risks to susceptible individuals. In 1997 the Ministry of Agriculture, Fisheries and Food (MAFF) launched an awareness campaign for caterers. The food industry as a whole is keen to assist, including food manufacturers (e.g. Heinz, Kinnerton, Nestlé), food retailers (e.g. Iceland, Sainsbury, Tesco), food outlets (e.g. McDonald's, Pret à Manger) and the catering industry (e.g. restaurants, canteens). They are making many positive changes to their practices and labelling to minimise the risks of allergens reaching susceptible people.

The initiatives that have had a positive impact on consumers include:

- Improved labelling on products, including 'May contain' notices.
- Many manufacturers ignoring the 25% rule and labelling ingredients fully.
- The availability of 'free from' lists.
- New production and distribution practices at manufacturer and retailer levels.
- Manufacturers of new special-diet products.
- Specific allergen labelling on food (e.g. 'suitable for a nut-free diet').
- Increased range of foods available.

There are, however, a number of legal, practical and commercial issues that cause complications at all of these levels of food production, distribution and consumption.

THE FOOD AND DRINK FEDERATION

The Food and Drink Federation produces *Food Allergen Advice Notes*, which provides advice for manufacturers on the identification and control of major food allergens and on consumer information. The allergens include peanuts, tree nuts, fish, shellfish, cow's milk, eggs, soya beans and sesame seeds. These advice notes cover:

- Definitions and lists of allergens.
- Consumer information.
- Good allergy practice, such as:
  – information to staff,

– scrutiny of raw material/ingredients (including compound materials purchased from suppliers) to ensure that they are indeed free from the excluded items – e.g. the oats for a milk-free flapjack have not been coated in yoghurt or margarine,
– new product development,
– operational controls,
– monitoring clean-up procedures.

Detailed examples of good manufacturing practice include:

- Ensuring that raw materials are free from allergens by auditing and working with suppliers to prevent cross-contamination on suppliers' sites and during suppliers' production processes.
- Storing allergenic ingredients in specific areas that are clearly identified, and, where appropriate, using dedicated equipment to handle them. Colour coding is a good way of identifying these items.
- Scheduling production where equipment and personnel are used to manufacture several products, including some containing allergenic compounds. For example, manufacturing non-allergenic products first and allergenic products at the end of a production run; or, whenever possible, minimising changeovers by undertaking long runs of allergenic products followed by a major clean-down.

Copies of the *Food Allergens Advice Notes* are available, on request, from the Food and Drink Federation (for contact details, see Appendix 1).

THE FOOD STANDARDS AGENCY

The Food Standards Agency came into being on 3 April 2000. Before this it operated as the Joint Food Safety and Standards Group, which was mainly an amalgamation of departments in the Ministry of Agriculture, Fisheries and Food and the Department of Health that dealt with matters relating to food and food safety.

There are three main groups in the Food Standards Agency, which incorporates a range of specialist divisions set up to fulfil the Agency's roles and responsibilities.

Of these three groups, the Food Safety Policy Group deals with all aspects of food safety and nutrition. Much of this was previously split between the Ministry of Agriculture, Fisheries and Food and the Department of Health.

In the Food Safety Policy Group are eight divisions. The one that is pertinent to food allergy issues is the Chemical Safety and Toxicology Division. The aims of this Division are:

- to determine the limits of chemicals in food through the development of risk assessments,
- to develop policies and to advise about food allergies and the safety of natural toxicants,
- to ensure that consumer issues are taken into account in the safety assessments of pesticides and veterinary medicines.

TRADING STANDARDS

Trading Standards officers are responsible for enforcing food-labelling laws. They should be contacted if a food is labelled incorrectly – for example, if you have an allergic reaction to a food that, according to the ingredients label, is safe for you. The Trading Standards officer will obtain a sample of the product and analyse it in the laboratory to check for an undeclared ingredient on the label – based on your evidence.

SUPERMARKET FOOD-ALLERGEN LABELLING

Many supermarkets now have a labelling policy that is designed to help people with an allergy to read food labels. Customers are able to see at a glance whether products are suitable for a particular diet. For example, cow's-milk-free, nut-free, egg-free and wheat-free. The information is often in a panel or box, as part of the food labelling. It sometimes contains an easy-to-spot graphic such as an ear of corn to indicate that the product is suitable for a gluten-free diet, or a cow with a cross through it to indicate that the product is suitable for a cow's-milk-free diet.

'Free from' lists

All major supermarkets and many food manufacturers now voluntarily hold detailed lists of own-brand products that are free from all the major allergens, such as milk, nuts or eggs. They will even some-times compile a tailor-made list if you have more than one allergy. The supermarket head office or in-store customer services section will be able to advise you about this.

The 'free from' lists are an excellent guide, but you must always read the food labels as well to be sure that the foods are indeed safe for you.

THE FOOD INTOLERANCE DATABANK

The Food Intolerance Databank is a database of a range of food prod-ucts that are free from common food allergens, but it can be accessed only by a dietitian. Annually updated 'free from' lists of these are available through your dietitian (there may be a charge).

FOOD OUTLETS

At present there is no legal requirement for any catering outlet to give information about what has gone into the food on sale. However, many fast-food outlets now produce information on food ingredients. For example, McDonald's produces and has readily available a full ingredients listing for every product it sells.

Some fast-food outlets also keep food items separate from one another. Again, McDonald's have separate food preparation and cooking areas for each product. This considerably reduces the risk of cross-contamination (see Chapter 15) and, if you decide to eat out, it would be safer for you to eat in places that follow this practice. For more information about eating out, see Chapter 14 ('Eating Away from Home').

COSMETICS LABELLING

The sixth amendment to the European Union Cosmetic Directive (1993) was implemented in December 1997. It requires the ingredi-ents to be included in the label for soaps, cosmetics and 'personal care products'. This classification is taken to include any preparation that is applied to the skin, eyes, mouth, hair or nails for the purpose of cleansing, giving a pleasant smell or enhancing appearance. The labelling has helped consumers to identify products that might be harmful to them. However, because the labelling is in Latin, it is sometimes incomprehensible to the layperson. This can cause a problem when common ingredients are not recognised. An example of this is 'arachis oil', which is the International Nomenclature of Cosmetic Ingredients (INCI) name for peanut oil.

The only answer is for you to have a list with the Latin names of the ingredients that you must avoid and refer to this whenever buying products.

The Cosmetic Toiletry and Perfumery Association Ltd is prepared to answer queries about these issues and has a useful leaflet listing some of the Latin (INCI) names. Below is a list of some of the ordinary names and their Latin names.

Ingredients and their INCI names (as used on product packaging)

Ingredient	INCI name
Avocado	*Persea gratissima*
Bitter almond	*Prunus amara*
Brazil nut	*Bertholletia excelsa*
Coconut	*Cocos nucifera*
Cod liver oil	*Gadi iecur*
Egg	*Ovum*
Hazel nut	*Corylus rostrata/americana/avellana*
Macadamia nut	*Macademia ternifolia*
Melon	*Cucumis melo*
Milk	*Lac*
Mixed fish oil	*Piscum iecur*
Pea	*Pisum sativum*
Peanut oil	Arachis oil
Sesame	*Sesamum indicum*
Soya	*Glycine soja*

Ingredient	INCI name
Sweet almond/Almond oil	*Prunus dulcis*
Walnut	*Juglans regia/nigra*

A comprehensive inventory of these substances has been published by the European Commission and is available on their website or on the Cosmetic Toiletry and Perfumery Association website (see Appendix 2).

The terminology used in the labelling of these products must comply with that in the inventory.

GUIDANCE ON FOOD-LABELLING RULES

Notes giving informal guidance about the food-labelling rules, and on issues raised by them, have been produced by MAFF (see Appendix 1 for contact details). Notes on the following subjects are available, free of charge:

- the Food Labelling Regulations 1996,
- nutrition labelling,
- nutrition claims,
- quantitative ingredient declarations (QUID),
- labelling of foods that contain genetically modified soya or maize,
- labelling of alcoholic drinks,
- which foods should carry a 'use by' date.

Guidelines on products for people with an allergy

The Local Authorities Co-ordinating Body on Foods and Trading Standards (LACOTS) has created guidelines on the use of the terms 'non-allergic', 'hypo-allergenic' and 'allergy-free'. There are currently no standard definitions, so the terms can be misleading and need clarification. LACOTS has stated that all products have the potential to cause an allergic reaction, and therefore all three terms are potentially misleading. In a bid to standardise the terminology, LACOTS has suggested that the term 'hypo-allergenic' is more correct, as it indicates that every effort has been made to reduce a product's allergenic potential.

GENETICALLY MODIFIED (GM) FOODS AND ALLERGIES

A study published in 1996 found that soya beans genetically engineered with a gene from Brazil nuts could trigger a reaction in people with an allergy to Brazil nuts. This study has become well known and is often cited as one reason why GM foods may increase the risk of allergies.

WARNING

A friend who is severely allergic to milk recently decided to indulge in some chocolate that was labelled as vegan/dairy-free. The label was obviously wrong because she had a severe anaphylactic reaction and had to be rushed to hospital. This is a very rare occurrence but it highlights how important it is, if you have a severe allergy, *always* to carry your adrenaline with you.

10
Special Diets

The major sections in this chapter have information and advice about specific special diets. They also advise how to follow the diets accurately and how to prevent nutritional deficiencies by adding replacement foods into your diet.

Some people think that they are already following a special diet and totally avoiding a particular food allergen, when they are actually eating components of that allergen without knowing it. For example, a person severely allergic to milk might not be aware that biscuits, muesli and sweets may contain derivatives of milk that are sufficient to cause a severe reaction. (This may account for allergic reactions of 'unknown origin'.) The main reason for this is that there is often a poor awareness of food allergen derivatives that are present in an ingredient but labelled with a different name. (Food labelling is discussed in Chapter 9.) A dietitian will be able to help you recognise these names, and thus avoid them.

Having to give up a particular food may not be as disastrous as you might first think. There may even be some positive changes to your diet, such as new recipe ideas and the chance to experiment with new foods. Your culinary skills may be desperate to get out – so now is their chance! Even if you hate cooking, there are still lots of ways that you can enjoy your food – this chapter will give you some ideas. However, the changes do mean taking responsibility for your own diet. You can no longer just accept the food that is offered when you eat out without discussing your requirements with your host or the restaurant staff.

There is no substitute for a full assessment by a dietitian (see Chapter 8), who will advise you on appropriate food substitutes. This is especially important if you have more than one allergy, because exclusion of many foods is likely to leave you with an unbalanced diet. The dietitian will also advise you about cross-contamination issues (discussed in Chapter 15). To see a dietitian, you need a referral from your GP or hospital specialist. This is the case whether the dietitian is part of the NHS or in private practice.

The websites listed in Appendixes 1 and 2 will help you find up-to-date information about products for special diets. They will help in your pursuit of a safe environment for enjoying food and socialising without the worry of cross-contamination – forever! Appendix 3 has details of useful books and Appendix 1 has a section giving details of safe restaurant and accommodation choices. See also Chapters 13 ('Eating In'), 14 ('Eating Away from Home') and 16 ('Holidays and Travelling').

DAIRY-FREE DIET

What exactly are dairy foods? There is, in fact, a lot of confusion about the term 'dairy'. Essentially, it is *cow's milk and its derivatives*: cow's milk, cream, butter, cheese and related items such as yoghurt, fromage frais and dairy ice-cream. Many processed foods contain dairy products. The obvious foods such as milk chocolate and rice pudding are easy to avoid but the 'hidden' sources of milk (e.g. *casein* and *whey*) can cause confusion and sometimes inadvertent allergic reactions.

Below is a list of dairy components to be avoided when on a dairy-free diet. By reading labels closely, it should be possible for you to avoid them.

- butter, butter oil, buttermilk,
- casein, caseinates, hydrolysed casein, sodium caseinate,
- cheese,
- cow's milk (fresh, UHT, evaporated, condensed, dried),
- cream,
- curd,
- ghee,
- lactic acid (E270),
- lactoglobulin,
- lactose,
- milk solids,
- whey, hydrolysed whey, whey powder, whey syrup sweetener,
- yoghurt, fromage frais.

'Flavourings' may contain any of the above ingredients. Strictly speaking, lactose is milk sugar and does not contain allergenic proteins. However, some people who are allergic to milk report reactions to it, which suggests that there is a chance that it can be 'contaminated' with milk protein. Lactic acid may be derived from the process of fermenting milk or from the fermentation of pickles, cocoa or tobacco!

WHAT ABOUT GOAT'S, SHEEP'S AND EWE'S MILK?

Technically these are not dairy products. However, they have a similar composition to cow's milk and may cause allergic reactions similar to those caused by cow's milk.

REPLACEMENT FOODS AND INGREDIENTS

As with any special diet, you can make it more appealing by using replacement ingredients and special products.

Instead of	Choose
Butter	Soya or milk-free margarine
Cheese	Soya, rice, tofu cheese
Cow's milk	Soya, rice, oat, nut, pea protein milk
Cream	Soya cream, oat cream, coconut milk
Cream cheese	Soya cream cheese
Ice-cream	Soya ice-cream, oat ice-cream
Yoghurt	Soya yoghurt, oat yoghurt

Recipes for home-made soya milks can be found in any vegan cookbook. Alternatively, try making your own nut milks. For useful recipe books, see Appendix 3.

The end of this section gives lists of alternative or replacement products you can try. They were correct at the time of writing but remember *always* to read the labels *every* time you make a purchase, to check that they are still suitable.

DAIRY-FREE DIET AND NUTRITION

By using the replacement foods listed above you will be able to achieve adequate nutrition from your dairy-free diet. However, a dairy-free diet without these replacement foods is likely to be nutritionally deficient. It is always advisable to seek advice from a dietitian before you remove foods from your diet, especially staple foods such as milk. (Chapter 8 discusses how to get a referral to a dietitian.)

Calcium

Dairy foods are usually the main source of calcium in your diet, which is essential for the development of strong bones and teeth, normal blood clotting, nerve function and enzyme activity. It is especially important in children and adolescents but is in fact an essential nutrient throughout life. Women who are breast-feeding have a very high requirement. It is thought that adequate calcium in early life may help protect against osteoporosis (brittle bones) later on.

Daily calcium requirements

Age group	Calcium requirements
0–1 year	525mg
1–3 years	350mg
4–6 years	450mg
7–10 years	550mg
Males 11–18 years	1,000 mg
Males 19+ years	700 mg
Females 11–18 years	800 mg
Females 19+ years	700 mg

A woman who is breast-feeding requires an extra 550mg

Calcium content of common dairy-free calcium-rich foods in the diet

Food and average portion size	Calcium content
100g fried whitebait	860mg
100g cooked spinach	600mg
100g tofu (soya bean curd)	510mg
100g black treacle	500mg
100g sardines (if bones eaten)	500mg
100g dried figs	280mg
200ml calcium-enriched soya milk*	275mg
100g almonds	250mg
100g watercress	220mg
100g muesli	200mg
100g Brazil nuts	180mg
25g sunflower seeds	178mg
25g sesame seeds	160mg
100g red kidney beans	140mg
30g soya cheese	125mg
125g soya yoghurt	125mg
100g marzipan	120mg
100g white bread	100mg
60g shelled prawns	90mg
1 medium-sized orange	75mg
100g baked beans	50mg

* The amount of calcium in soya milk varies; it will be listed on the product label

To ensure that you have an adequate intake of calcium, make use of the replacement foods available. Also take other sources of calcium such as white and brown bread, dark green vegetables, canned fish (including the bones), baked beans and other pulses, nuts, seeds, dried fruit and muesli. Many commercial breakfast cereals are fortified with calcium, as are some fruit juices.

Vitamin D, which is manufactured in the body by the action of sunlight on the skin, and obtained from a variety of foods, helps with the absorption of calcium. Smoking and excess alcohol reduce its absorption.

For advice on calcium requirements, contact your local dietitian or obtain a leaflet from your local health authority's Health Promotion Team. (The number can be found in your local telephone directory.) Further information can be obtained from the National Osteoporosis Society (see Appendix 1) or a dietitian.

'Calciyums' are high-calcium biscuits designed especially for people on a dairy-free diet as an alternative source of calcium. They are available only in the USA at present, so ask a friend to get you some next time they are there!

Kosher food

Kosher, also known as 'parev' or 'pareve', food is usually dairy-free. This may increase the number of foods that are suitable for you on your dairy-free diet. Rakusen's and Snowcrest (Tofutti) are just two companies specialising in kosher foods.

Wine

Some wines (red, white and rosé) contain casein, which is used as a clarifying agent. Occasionally, minute traces can remain in the finished product, which are legally undeclared on the label.

Sex

It may be useful to know that most condoms contain casein, which is one of the main proteins in milk. If you are very sensitive to traces of milk, this may cause a problem, so beware! Casein-free condoms (Condomi Condoms) can be purchased from the Vegan Society.

Medication

- Many tablets contain lactose, which is a milk sugar. Lactose may cause an allergic reaction if you are severely allergic to milk, although most people with cow's milk allergy do not react to lactose.
- Lactose does not dissolve in water, so water-soluble tablets are generally free from lactose, but do check this with your pharmacist.
- It has been known for GPs to prescribe medication containing lactose to people with a milk allergy – including antihistamines that contain lactose to treat a reaction caused by milk! *Never assume* that your GP has remembered to prescribe medication that is lactose-free or that the ingredients are still the same. *Always check and be safe*. Check *every time* with your pharmacist, who will hold this information or will be happy to make some enquiries on your behalf.

Toiletries and cosmetics

Toiletries and cosmetics may contain cow's milk derivatives. See Chapter 9 ('Food Labelling') to find out how you can identify these products.

Sweeteners

Sweeteners may contain lactose. Remember to check the ingredients of the sweeteners offered to you, whether in granulated or in tablet form.

'Whiteners' in tea and coffee

Some milk alternatives tend to separate or curdle when added to tea or coffee. Cooling the drink a little first sometimes reduces this. Look in a vegan cookbook for information on how you can prevent this, or alternatively do some experiments of your own!

Glucono delta lactone

This is a form of sugar found in grapes, and is commonly used in breadmaking when yeast has to be avoided. Although the name is deceiving, it *does not* contain lactose.

SOME ALTERNATIVE OR REPLACEMENT FOODS

The information that follows is only a guide. Always read all ingredients labels thoroughly. If you are in any doubt whether a product is suitable for your special diet, please contact the manufacturer.

Soya milks

Alpro	Strawberry-flavoured soya milk
Evernat	Organic soya milk powder
	Organic nut drinks: almond/hazelnut
Granose (Haldane Foods)	In a variety of sizes – calcium-enriched; organic; sweetened or unsweetened
	Mini-milks: banana; chocolate; strawberry
Granovita	Sweetened and unsweetened; with added calcium; chocolate-flavoured; concentrated
healthfood shops	Own-brand soya milks
Heinz	With added calcium; vanilla flavoured
Plamil	Sweetened or unsweetened; with added calcium; with added vitamins; concentrated
Prosoya	*So Nice*: a range of plain and flavoured soya milks
Provamel	Sweetened and unsweetened; flavoured mini-milks: chocolate or vanilla or strawberry; with added calcium; with added vitamins
SoGood	Flavoured milks: chocolate or vanilla with added calcium and vitamins
Sojasun	Calcium-enriched sweetened soya milk or natural soya milk
Suma Wholefoods	Soya milk powder
Sunrise (Soya Health Foods)	Sweetened and unsweetened or flavoured soya drinks: banana; chocolate; strawberry
	Soya milk powder
supermarkets	Own-brand sweetened or unsweetened; with added calcium
Ultrapharm (Allergycare)	Soya milkshake powder: banana; vanilla; strawberry; coconut
Unisoy Gold	Soya milk with added calcium
Vitasoy	Soya milks: carob supreme; creamy original; rich cocoa; vanilla delite

Other alternative milks

Bart Spices	*Coconut* milk
Blue Dragon Foods	Tinned *coconut* milk; fat-reduced *coconut* milk
Clearspring	*Imagine* puddings: Rice Dream – *rice* drink: organic original; vanilla; chocolate; carob; calcium enriched
	Range includes lunchbox size: original; chocolate; vanilla
Evernat	Organic *almond* drink; organic *hazelnut* drink
First Foods	Organic *rice* drink
Lima	*Rice* drink: original; vanilla; chocolate
Plamil Foods	*White Sun*: *pea* protein alternative to milk; sweetened or non-sweetened
Provamel	*Rice* drink
Skane Dairy	Millmilk *oat* drink: original; chocolate; vanilla; fibre; organic
Ultrapharm (Allergycare)	*Rice* milk powder
Vitariz	Organic *rice* drink

'Creams'

Blue Dragon Foods	Creamy coconut
Granose (Haldane Foods)	Long-life Soya Creem
Provamel	Soya Dream
Rich's	Whip topping
Snowcrest (Tofutti)	Big Top pareve (no meat or dairy products) cream whip
SoGood	UHT soya cream
Sojami (Organic Supplies)	Dairy-free soya-based vegan crème fraîche

'Cheese' and 'cheese' spreads

Bute Island Foods	*Scheese* (hard 'cheese'): Cheddar/Cheddar with chives; Cheshire; Edam; Gouda; hickory Cheddar; mozzarella; stilton; emmentale
Fayrefield Foods	*Winner Swedish Soft*: non-dairy, non-animal equivalent to full-fat soft cheese: plain; garlic and herb
First Foods	Oat-based dairy-free cream cheese

Galaxy Foods	Soya cheese slices: Cheddar; mozzarella. **Beware** of the *rice cheese slices*, because they contain casein
Kallo Foods	*Fromsoya* – soya cheese spreads: original; garlic; dill; onion
La Font Della Vita	Vegan cheese alternative
Morehands Ltd	*Florentino* – Parmazano: a non-animal dairy/milk/egg-free parmesan style
Plas Farm	'Cheese' spreads: coriander and lemon; plain; garlic and herb. Hard 'cheese': *Vegerella* – Biddy Merkins cheese substitute; Italian/Mexican
Redwood	*Cheezly*, tofu cheese: red Cheddar; white Cheddar; barbecue style; garlic and parsley; pizza style
Soderasens	*Fromsoya*: dill; horseradish and lemon; onion; garlic, parsley and onion
Tofutti	*Better than cream cheese*: French onion; plain; garlic and herbs; chives and herbs
Whole Earth	*Soya Kaas*: Cheddar; mozzarella

Note that several other soya cheeses of US origin (e.g. Rice Parmesan, Light & Less, Rice Slice and Soya Kaas) are designed for the low-fat market rather than the dairy-free market. As a result, to improve their consistency they include *casein* – which is a milk protein – making them unsuitable for a dairy-free diet.

'Cheese flavouring'

Nutritional yeast-flakes are a product made from molasses and produced specifically for the healthfood market. It is a yellow flake with a sweet cheesy taste, and is excellent as flavouring for cheese-type sauces. It can also be used as a topping sprinkled on lasagne or pizza or mixed with mashed potato and cooked in the oven as cheese and potato bake. The flakes can also be mixed with a dairy-free margarine to be spread on bread and toasted under the grill.

Engevita Nutritional Flakes from Marigold Healthfoods are available from most healthfood shops. Alternatively, *The Uncheese Cookbook* (see Appendix 3) contains recipes for you to make your own dairy-free cheese.

Pesto

| Suma | Vegan pesto |
| G Costa & Co. Ltd | *Zest Foods*: vegan pesto; vegan gluten-free pesto; sun-dried tomato paste |

Some dairy-free margarines

	Milk-free	Soya-free	Corn-free	Rape-free	Nut/peanut-free	Palm nut-free	Coconut-free
Biona *							
Olive Extra	Yes	Yes	Yes	Yes	Yes	Yes	Yes
Organic Veg	Yes	No	Yes	Yes	Yes	Yes	Yes
Organic Veg	Yes	Yes	Yes	No	Yes	Yes	Yes
Pure †							
Sunflower	Yes	Yes	Yes	Yes	Yes	No	Yes
Soya	Yes	No	Yes	Yes	Yes	No	Yes
Organic	Yes	No	Yes	Yes	Yes	No	Yes
Suma							
Sunflower	Yes	Yes	Yes	Yes	Yes	No	Yes
Soya	Yes	No	Yes	Yes	Yes	No	Yes
Tomor ‡	Yes	No	Yes	Yes	Yes	Yes	No
Vitaquell	Yes	Yes	No	Yes	Yes	No	Yes
Whole Earth	Yes	No	Yes	Yes	Yes	No	Yes

*Windmill Organics; † Matthews Foods; ‡ Rakusen's

Margarine/Fat

Windmill Organics	*Biona*: extra virgin olive oil organic dairy-free spread; soya-free; dairy-free; vegan
	Organic sunflower vegetable spread free from dairy/milk products and their derivatives; vegan
Flora	White Flora
Granose (Haldane Foods)	Soya margarine; sunflower margarine; diet half-fat spread; olive grove margarine; low-salt vegetable margarine

Granovita	Non-hydrogenated sunflower margarine; non-hydrogenated low-fat spread
Matthews Foods	*Pure*: sunflower margarine; soya spread
Meridian Foods	Soya margarine
Rakusen's	*Tomor*: block margarine; sunflower tubs
Smilde Food Group	Sunflower spread
Suma Wholefoods	Low-fat spread; soya spread; 100% sunflower spread; organic spread
supermarkets	Own-brands of soya margarines; dairy-free low-fat spreads
Vitaquell	Margarine selection: organic; extra; cuisine; light

'Yoghurts'

First Foods	Oat-based dairy-free yoghurts in various flavours
Granose (Haldane Foods)	Soya yoghurts: apricot; blackcurrant and apple; peach melba; strawberry
Granovita	*Deluxe Soyage* non-dairy cultured soya dessert: peach and apricot; raspberry; strawberry; natural; black cherry
	Soyage Organic: strawberry; peach; forest fruits
Haldane Foods	*SoGood* non-dairy cultured yoghurt: black cherry; peach and passion fruit; strawberry; pineapple; natural. Gluten-free, milk-free, egg-free, animal-free
	Yoga organic dairy-free yoghurts: blueberry; peach and apricot; plain; strawberry
Linda McCartney	*Dairy-Like Yoga*: various flavours
NGT Associates	*Yosa*: dairy- and soya-free desserts: fruits of the forest; peach and passionfruit; pineapple; apple and banana – all with added calcium
Provamel	Strawberry; peach; black cherry; red cherry; peach and mango; vanilla; plain
	Yofu Junior for children: strawberry and banana; peach and pear
Prosoya	*So Nice Soyog*: strawberry; peach; forest fruit; raspberry
SoGood	Natural; peach and passion fruit; black cherry; strawberry; pineapple
Sojasun	Natural; apricot and guava; raspberry and passion fruit
Unisoy	Raspberry; black cherry; peach melba

Non-frozen desserts

Clearspring	*Imagine* puddings: banana; butterscotch; chocolate; lemon
Organic Valley	Organic dairy-free rice pudding
Plamil	Non-dairy soya desserts: Pots: chocolate; vanilla; hazelnut. Cartons: vanilla and chocolate. Rice pudding with sultanas: sweetened or unsweetened
Provamel	Organic soya desserts: Cartons: vanilla; chocolate Pots: vanilla; chocolate; hazelnut
Sojasun	Non-dairy dessert: vanilla; chocolate

'Ice-creams'

First Foods	Oat-based dairy-free ice-cream: vanilla; strawberry; chocolate
Haldane Foods	*Ice Delight* organic frozen non-dairy soya dessert: strawberry swirl; chocolate swirl
Linda McCartney	Soya-based frozen dessert: strawberry dream; vanilla toffee; double chocolate
Maranelli's	*Soya Supreme Dessert*: chocolate; vanilla; raspberry ripple
Provamel	Single tubs and 1 litre: strawberry; vanilla; chocolate; fudge
Soya Health Foods	*Sunrise*: soya-based carob-chocolate ice Non-dairy *Ice Dream*: raspberry ripple; vanilla; chocolate
Fayrefield Foods	*Winner Swedish Glace*: 1 litre: strawberry; raspberry; vanilla; chocolate; mocha and chocolate ripple Cone: strawberry ripple Lolly Tots: alternative to luxury ice-cream on a stick: vanilla; strawberry
Tofutti	Individual tubs: vanilla fudge Large tubs: butter pecan; chocolate cookie; chocolate supreme; vanilla fudge; madagascan vanilla; wildberry supreme Cones: vanilla and pecan nut Ice cake: Rock 'n' Roll (similar to Vienetta)

Chocolate

Animal Aid	Selection of non-dairy boxes and bars of chocolate
Benedicts	Chocolate ginger
Buxton Foods	*The Stamp collection*: dairy-free chocolates: sultana; apricot; sunflower seed
Choconat	Dark chocolate and almonds; organic; plain organic
Devon Fudge Direct	Chocolate flavoured
Doves Farm	Chocolate chip cookies; plain chocolate digestives
Dr Hadwen Trust	Selection of handmade non-dairy vegan chocolates: chocolate Brazils; cherry liqueurs; assortments; mint creams; chocolate ginger; gold selection; chocolate animals; etc.
Fry's (Cadbury)	Chocolate cream bars: orange; peppermint; mint
Granny Ann (Itona)	Beanmilk chunky eggs
Granovita	Chocolate spread; range of milk-free chocolates
Jeanette	Chunky nut brittle dark; dark chocolate hazelnut and raisins; vegan assortment
Lindt	Excellence, Surfin and Thin bars
Lyme Regis Foods	Chocolate marzipan bar; variety of carob bars
Nestlé Rowntree	*After Eight*: dark chocolate version
Norfolk Truffle Co	Dairy-free organic range of truffles: 10 flavours
Plamil	*Expressions* non-dairy milk chocolate; organic dark; organic orange; organic mint dark
	Non-dairy carob bars: plain; hazelnut; orange; no added sugar; no added sugar drops
	Martello non-dairy milk chocolate; dark plain; hazelnut; mint
	Carob spread: sweetened; unsweetened
Rapunzel (Windmill Organic)	Swiss chocolate: plain organic; plain with almonds organic
Ricci	Carob-coated chocolate bars: coconut; lime; orange
Shepherd Boy	*Just So* carob bars: crispy; orange; peppermint; ginger; fruit and nut
Suma	Carob drops
supermarkets	Own-brands. Various – see their 'free from' lists

Sweet Temptation	Carob products: boxed Easter eggs; boxed teddy; box of bunnies; mini-eggs with surprise inside Carob bars: original; mint; orange
Thornton's	Various: details on their 'free from' list
Tropical Source (Community Foods)	Chocolate in bars: toasted almond; Californian raisin and currant; hazelnut expresso crunch; wild rice crisp; red raspberry crush; candy mint crunch
Ultrapharm	*Allergycare*. Whizzers: dairy-free chocolate: chocolate beans; footballs; mint balls; speckled eggs; toffees; mint toffee humbugs Silhouette carob bar original Dairy-free real chocolate spread
Vegan Society	Fine mint chocolates; organic gourmet chocolate truffles
Viva!	Selection of dairy-free bars and boxes of chocolates
Whole Earth Foods	*Green & Black's* organic dairy-free chocolate: organic dark; dark hazelnut and currant; Maya gold Dairy-free Easter egg wrapped in foil in a presentation box

The replacement products listed above are found mainly in health-food shops, but supermarkets are increasingly stocking a selection. If you have any problems finding them in your area, contact the manufacturer or distributor (listed in Appendix 1) for details of stockists near you, or you may be able to order them through your healthfood shop or by mail order.

EGG-FREE DIET

EGG ALLERGY

The main proteins responsible for egg allergy are present in the egg white but some of the proteins in egg yolk may also induce an allergic response. Avoid eggs from all birds, because they are similar in chemical structure and therefore are likely to trigger similar allergic reactions.

Cooking eggs 'denatures' many of the egg proteins, which means that some people can tolerate cooked eggs even if they are allergic to raw eggs. Despite this, if you have a severe allergy that is likely to trigger an anaphylactic reaction to one form of egg, you should avoid all eggs in all forms.

Is it safe to eat chicken and other poultry?

Yes! This is because the proteins in the flesh of the birds are different from those in the eggs.

FOODS CONTAINING EGGS

It is relatively easy to avoid eggs if they are served on their own. However, they are often a 'hidden' or 'disguised' ingredient in prepared and manufactured foods.

Whether you are planning to eat foods prepared by yourself or by others, it is essential that you understand all the names that egg derivatives or components can be called:

Albumin	Dried egg	Ovoglobulin
Egg (all bird eggs)	Frozen egg	Ovomucin
Egg powder	Globulin	Ovovitellin
Egg protein	Lecithin (E322)	Pasteurised egg
Egg white	Livetin	Ovomucin
Egg yolk	Ovalbumin	Vitellin

Theoretically, lecithin can be derived from egg, but in practice this is rare. Where egg lecithin does appear, it is likely to be in medicinal products but this is by no means common. Your pharmacist should be able to supply information about any medicines you are prescribed. Soya lecithin is egg-free.

Other important points are:

- Always read the food ingredient label to see if it contains egg in any form. If the food does not have a label (such as bakery goods), *do not* eat it. (See Chapter 9 for information about how to understand and read food labels.)
- Understand cross-contamination issues (see Chapter 15).
- Eat only foods that you are completely sure are safe to eat.
- To add variety to your diet when you cannot eat eggs you can use existing recipes, but with whole egg-replacer instead of whole egg, and egg white replacer instead of egg white. (Some common replacements for egg are listed at the end of this section.)
- Substitute eggs with something else, depending on their purpose in the recipe: leavening agent, raising agent, glazing agent, binding agent, source of liquid. The Table below shows alternatives, according to the usual function of the egg in the recipe:

Purpose of egg in recipe	Substitute
Leavening	15ml (1 tbsp) baking powder + 30ml (2 tbsp) liquid
Glazing	Sugar and water or gelatine glaze
Binding (1 egg =)	Soya milk; soya dessert; custard; mashed banana; soya cream; white sauce 50g (1¾ oz) tofu; *or* 100ml (⅓ cup) water + 5ml (1 tsp) arrowroot powder + 10ml (2 tsp) guar gum
Liquid (1 egg =)	100ml (⅓ cup) apple juice; 15ml (1 tbsp) vinegar; 60ml (4 tbsp) pureed apricot
Raising agent (1 egg =)	15ml (1 tbsp) baking powder; 3.75ml (¾ tsp) bicarbonate of soda + 10ml (2 tsp) cider vinegar

- Try some recipes that are egg-free. These may be recipes that just happen to be egg-free or they may be from a vegan or special-diet cookbook (see Appendix 3), or those supplied with the egg replacer.

- Request a 'free from egg' list from the supermarket(s) where you shop. This is a list of all their own-brand products that are free from egg. It is a free service, but you may have to ask the supermarket's head office for the list.
- Request a 'free from egg' list from your favourite manufacturers (e.g. Walkers, Findus).
- Make use of foods manufactured specifically for people allergic to eggs (e.g. egg-free nougat and egg-free cakes).
- Buy vegan foods, as they are always egg-free.
- Eat out in a vegan or special-diet restaurant or go to a vegan guesthouse or one that caters specifically for special diets. As well as enjoying the treat, it will allow you access to lots of other recipe ideas; you may be able to chat to the chef and look at his or her cookbook selection if you ask nicely!

Tales of the un*egg*spected ...

Below are examples of items that you might never have guessed could contain egg:

- some medicines,
- consommé soup (egg is used as a clarifier),
- hair shampoo and conditioner,
- icing and icing flowers,
- nutritional supplements (e.g. vitamin and mineral preparations),
- pet foods,
- some fur garments,
- some photographic film,
- some printed natural fabrics that have not yet been washed,
- some wines and champagnes (egg albumen can be used as a clarifying agent),
- vaccinations grown on an egg culture (although it is unlikely that the vaccine will be contaminated by egg, it is probably better to be safe than sorry).

Note The Vegan Society and most supermarkets selling own-brands can provide a list of wines and champagnes that have not been clarified with egg. Alternatively, buy from a vegan wine merchant. There are two major independent merchants in the UK selling vegan wine direct to customers by mail order and to shops and restaurants: Vintage Roots Ltd and Vinceremos Wines & Spirits (contact details in Appendix 1). Healthfood shops are another source of vegan wines.

MEASLES, MUMPS AND RUBELLA (MMR) VACCINE

The MMR vaccine contains live measles virus that may be cultured on chick embryo cells, but it is unlikely that the vaccine is contaminated by egg protein. It is extremely unlikely that this vaccine could cause a reaction in an egg-allergic individual but make sure that the doctor knows about your child's allergy. If necessary, a skin-prick test using the vaccine can be done first. If this shows no reaction, the vaccine can be given safely. Both the skin-prick test and the vaccination should be done in hospital.

It is very important that you do not prevent your child from having the MMR vaccination. The risks from these three diseases are much greater than from a possible allergic reaction.

ALTERNATIVES FOR EGGS

Substitute for	Name of product	Made by
Whole egg	Whole Egg Replacer	Cirrus Associates
	Ener-G Egg Replacer	General Dietary
	Loprofin Egg Replacer	Nutricia
	Egg Replacer	Ultrapharm (Allergycare)
Egg white	Rite-Diet Egg White Replacer	Nutricia
Egg yolk, egg white, or whole egg	No-Egg Replacer	Orgran

EGG-FREE FOODS

Alternative Cakes	Egg-free cakes (vegan): rich chocolate loaf-tin; coffee walnut loaf-tin
Annie's Naturals	Selection of salad dressings and vinaigrette
Avalon	Egg-free 'saladaise': plain; garlic; cajunaise
Blue Dragon	Egg-free whole-wheat noodles and rice noodles
G Costa & Co. Ltd	Zest Foods Vegan pesto and vegan gluten-free pesto
Fabulous Foods	The Noodle Co. Egg-free noodles: chilli and garlic; spinach
Granovita	Egg-free mayonnaise: plain; lemon; garlic
manufacturers	Obtain their 'free from' list so that you can identify their egg-free products

Mrs Crimble's	Dutch fruit loaf free from egg and wheat
Orgran (Community Foods)	Sponge pudding mixes: chocolate; lemon
Plamil	Organic sandwich spreads: with paprika (soya-free); with tofu, curry and pineapple (gluten- and yeast-free); with vegetables (soya-free) Egg-free mayonnaise: garlic; plain; chilli; tarragon; organic
St Giles	*Duchesse.* Egg-free dressing and dips: garlic; tofu; dill pickle *Life, all natural products.* Egg-free salad cream; mayonnaise; tomato ketchup; brown sauce; Worcestershire sauce; tartare sauce; horseradish sauce
Suma	Vegannaise: plain; garlic. Vegan pesto: red; green
supermarkets	Own-brands: obtain their 'free from' lists so that their egg-free products can be identified
Village Bakery	Egg-free slices: date; apricot Cakes: fruit cake Fruit bars: nut; seed; fruit

PEANUT-FREE AND NUT-FREE DIETS

There has been a lot of publicity about peanut and nut allergies in recent years. This is because these allergies are becoming more common and also because a number of deaths related to peanut and nut allergy have been reported in the mass media.

Peanuts and nuts are often talked about as one and the same thing. They do not, however, belong to the same food family. Peanuts are legumes, which grow in the ground – so they are also known as groundnuts. They are from the *Leguminosae* plant family, which contains over 30 species, including peas, beans, lentils, soya beans, carob and liquorice. (For information about food families, see Chapter 12.) Some people who are allergic to peanuts are concerned that they may also be allergic to these other foods in this family. A report from the USA found that 5% of the children studied who had reacted to one legume had symptoms with multiple legumes. Nevertheless, if you are allergic to peanuts it is probably unnecessary to eliminate other legumes (such as peas, beans and lentils) from your diet unless there is good reason to suspect that they cause problems.

Botanically, peanuts are unrelated to tree nuts such as Brazil, macadamia, cashew, almond, walnut, pecan and hazelnut. However, it is fairly common for someone with peanut allergy to react to these as well. Whether you should avoid all nuts because you are allergic to peanuts, and vice-versa, is a question that cannot be answered, because the risk is not known. *Some* people with peanut allergy can eat tree nuts without a problem – allergy tests may help to determine this. If you have lived safely for many years without taking these precautionary measures, you could continue to do so but you will be taking a risk (perhaps you have just been lucky so far). If you have had an allergic reaction to any of them, though, it is generally recommended that you exclude all peanuts and all tree nuts from your diet.

It is usually wise to avoid eating anything with nuts until you have obtained advice from an allergy specialist. This is because peanuts are sometimes used as a cheap substitute for more expensive nuts, as they can be washed and treated to taste like almonds, walnuts or Brazil nuts. It has been known for an 'almond slice' to contain peanuts instead of almonds and for peanuts to be crushed and then re-formed into an almond shape for decorating chocolates or cakes. So *beware*!

Unfortunately, cooking nuts does not make them any less allergenic.

OTHER NAMES FOR PEANUT

As well as the Latin name, *Arachis hypogaea*, peanuts have several other names:

English	French	Dutch	Spanish
earth nut	arachide	aardnoot	cacahuete
goober nuts	cacahouette	aardnoten	
goober peas	caouette	apenoot	
groundnut	pistache de terre	olienoot	
mandalona nut	pinda (pindakaas)		
monkey-nut			

You can look up the names in other languages in a comprehensive dictionary, but don't assume you can correctly pronounce or understand the word when it is spoken. Alternatively, contact the British Allergy Foundation for a translation in most languages.

PEANUT DERIVATIVES

Hydrolysed vegetable protein, which is used to add flavour to foods, may cause an allergic reaction in an extremely sensitive person. The source is usually soya or wheat but it can be derived from peanut. The source does not have to be declared on the ingredients label, but some food manufacturers and retailers do so. If you are unsure whether the ingredient is safe, contact the manufacturer or retailer before you eat the food.

More obvious peanut derivatives are:

- arachis (peanut) oil (see below),
- peanut flour,
- peanut protein,
- unrefined peanut oil (see below).

Arachis oil is the International Nomenclature of Cosmetic Ingredients (INCI) name for peanut oil, and is often the name given in lists of ingredients.

PEANUT OIL

Peanut oil is also known as groundnut oil and arachis oil. It may be refined or unrefined.

The Seed Crushers and Oil Processors Association (SCOPA), of which all UK refiners of edible oil are members, funded research into the allergenicity of peanut oil. Its findings were published in 1997 in the *British Medical Journal*. The report concluded that **refined** peanut oil poses little or no risk to people with peanut allergy; in the unlikely event of a reaction, it would almost certainly be mild. Nevertheless, **unrefined** (crude) peanut oil should be avoided, because it may contain minute traces of peanut protein. The ultimate decision lies with you.

Following the research, SCOPA set up a code of practice to ensure that the presence of unrefined oil in a food product is always declared on the label. SCOPA also liaise with the Federation of European Oil Processors (also called FEDIOL) to persuade the EU to adopt this code of practice. The agreed code includes the following:

- SCOPA members selling unrefined peanut oil to the retail and wholesale food industry will state on the label 'contains unrefined peanut oil'.

- SCOPA members will obtain agreement from the retailer/ distributor that any food product that is made using this unrefined peanut oil will be labelled accordingly.
- SCOPA members selling unrefined peanut to the catering industry will declare 'unrefined peanut oil' on the label.
- SCOPA members will produce documentation that will advise the catering company buying the oil to declare the use of unrefined peanut oil to the consumer.

In summary, if a product contains unrefined peanut oil, it will be declared on the label. If a food contains refined peanut oil, it will only be declared if it is the only oil in a product; otherwise it will be included as 'vegetable oil' on the label. Both of these points apply only to foods manufactured in the UK or EU.

(For more details contact the Anaphylaxis Campaign for their fact-sheet on peanut oil.)

'MAY CONTAIN' WARNINGS ON FOOD LABELS

Food manufacturers and retailers have become increasingly allergy-aware over the past few years. They are striving to ensure that the public is informed about the food they eat. Because of cross-contamination issues (see Chapter 15), 'may contain' warnings have now been placed on many foods that do not themselves contain peanuts or nuts but may have become contaminated with traces of these foods. This has caused a lot of discontent among people with a peanut or nut allergy, because it has resulted in a vast restriction on the food now available to them. The positive side, however, is that you can be confident that the remaining foods should be safe for you to eat, and that being informed in this way means that you are not taking uncalculated risks. (See also Chapter 9, 'Food Labelling'.)

IS PEANUT OR NUT ALLERGY ON THE INCREASE?

Peanuts are now one of the main causes of food allergy reactions in the UK. Allergy clinics report an increase in the number of patients with peanut allergy, particularly in children. The exact reason for this is not known but it is suspected that a number of factors are involved (see Chapter 1). A major factor is the increased availability of peanuts in the British diet. This has led to increased exposure of babies (both in the womb and during breast-feeding) and young children to peanuts and peanut products and their proteins. Because the immune system (see Chapter 1) is not fully developed this early in life, such exposure seems to be one of the causes of the increased prevalence of nut and peanut allergies. More research is needed to determine whether this is true.

HOW DANGEROUS IS PEANUT/NUT ALLERGY?

The small number of reported deaths due to peanut and nut allergies are often from people in their teens and early twenties. This may be because they become more independent and are no longer protected by their parents much of the time and because they may not be as careful about keeping their medication with them at all times.

Compared with the everyday risks that we all take, such as travelling by car or crossing a busy road, death due to nut or peanut anaphylaxis is rare. However, if you also have asthma, the risk is greater. Even so, it is vital that we keep the problem in perspective; otherwise the allergy could become an all-consuming obsession.

REDUCING THE DANGER OF A SEVERE REACTION

Outgrowing the allergy
Some people (usually children) do outgrow a nut/peanut allergy. However, it is impossible to predict who will lose their allergy, and you should *never* try to test yourself. You should be properly assessed with skin-prick and RAST testing and then, if appropriate, with a carefully monitored 'oral challenge' – taking a suspect food by mouth (see also Chapter 2, 'Food Allergy Tests').

Desensitisation
Desensitisation is unsuitable for someone with a severe food allergy. It is discussed in Chapter 3 ('Will My Allergy Improve over Time?').

Vaccination
Vaccination against nut/peanut allergy is also discussed in Chapter 3.

Airline travel and nuts
The problems caused by nuts during air travel are discussed in Chapter 16 ('Holidays and Travelling').

Nut allergies and schools
See Chapter 6 for coping with food allergies when at school.

EATING OUT WITH A PEANUT/NUT ALLERGY

If you have a severe peanut/nut allergy and you want to eat out, you must be vigilant, ask all the right questions and, of course, carry your medication. Unless you have prepared the food yourself, you cannot be sure that it is completely safe.

If you decide that you are prepared to take this risk, the following suggestions will help to keep it to a minimum:

- Avoid Chinese, Thai, Malaysian and Indian restaurants. They use a lot of nuts and peanuts in their dishes, so there is a risk of cross-contamination (see Chapter 15).
- Use the same restaurant regularly, so that they become familiar with your needs.
- Go at a quiet time rather than when things are hectic and your needs might be unintentionally overlooked.
- Patronise a place that has a nut/peanut policy and general allergy-awareness. (Be wary of the MAFF 'Allergy aware' sticker, though. The restaurant might have changed hands and the present owners and staff do not know what the sticker implies.)
- Give the chef written guidelines about your needs, to prevent ambiguity. Ask that they be placed in a file for future use, or take a copy to the chef every time you are planning to eat in that restaurant or café.
- Choose simple dishes that are less likely to be contaminated.
- Telephone first, so that your meal can be made in advance and covered, ready to heat up later when the kitchen is busy.
- If you are not confident that your needs can be met but would like to join friends or colleagues who are eating out, ask if you can take your own ready-prepared food that can be heated up (or take a cold dish) and brought to you alongside the others' meals. Most places are more than happy for you to do this rather than risk taking responsibility for your food! (See also Chapter 14, 'Eating Away from Home'.)

Tales of the un*nut*spected!

Besides being a source of human nutrition, peanut and peanut products are used in animal and bird feeds and in skin creams. Under the European Union Cosmetic Directive, which came into force in December 1997, cosmetics products containing peanut oil must list the ingredients. The name used will probably be *Arachis hypogaea*. (See Chapter 9, 'Food Labelling', for more details.)

Traces of nuts and cross-contamination

Traces of peanuts or peanut dust can be inhaled when you are near someone who is eating them – such as when travelling by air, where peanut snacks are distributed with drinks – or where a large number of nuts are on display – as in a supermarket at Christmas time. Cross-contamination can also occur, and is discussed in Chapter 15.

POSSIBLE PEANUT DERIVATIVES

Carob Research suggests that carob is safe for people with peanut/nut allergy

Coconut and nutmeg Despite the word 'nut' in their names, coconut and nutmeg are not related to peanuts or nuts. An allergic reaction to either is unlikely but has been known to occur in a small number of individuals, including people with nut/peanut allergy. If you are concerned, NHS allergy clinics may do an allergy test if you ask for one.

E471 and E472 These are food additives that act as emulsifiers. It is technically possible, though highly unlikely, for E471 and E472 to be derived from peanut oil. Even if peanut oil was the source, the risk of an allergic reaction would be extremely low because the oil would have been refined.

Essence of nuts Although there have been no reported reactions to essence of nuts such as almond essence, you are advised to avoid them.

Lecithin Lecithin is an emulsifier, usually derived from unrefined soya oil or, very occasionally, from egg. In 1998, SCOPA (see earlier in this chapter) stated 'Lecithin is not derived from peanut oil'.

Palm nuts and pine nuts Palm nuts and pine nuts are not botanically related to peanuts or tree nuts but they may cause reactions in a small number of people. Caution is advised.

ALTERNATIVE PEANUT/NUT-FREE SWEETS

Peanut/nut-free chocolates

Kinnerton	Good range of peanut/nut-free chocolate made in the UK on a production line separate from peanut/nut varieties
Nestlé	Selection of peanut/nut-free chocolate made on a production line separate from their peanut/nut varieties
Vermont	Large selection of peanut/nut-free chocolates

Peanut/nut-free sweets

Sweets are easy to locate. Any 'free from' list will help you, and most packets are well labelled.

SESAME-FREE DIET

SESAME SEED ALLERGY

Sesame seeds are becoming increasingly popular in the UK. So is the small but significant number of people who are severely allergic to them. If you are allergic to sesame, you must avoid it completely – both in its cooked and in its uncooked form.

Sesame seeds are used extensively in the food industry, so it is important to read food labels carefully. Sesame can also be known as:

- anjoli/anjonjoli
- benne seeds/benne oil
- gingili/gingelly
- oleum
- *Sesamum indicum*
- simsim
- teel
- til

Sesamum indicum is the Latin name for sesame, and has been used in labelling on cosmetics, toiletries and perfumes since 1998. (See also Chapter 9 for more about food labelling.)

SESAME OIL

Sesame oil made from pulped ('cold pressing') sesame seeds is one of the few vegetable oils that can be used without being refined. This unrefined oil is likely to contain a significant amount of sesame seed protein, the part of the seed that can trigger an allergic reaction. If you have a sesame allergy, you must avoid all forms of sesame oil.

Because sesame seeds are very small, they are easily transferred by cross-contamination (see Chapter 15).

YOU SHOULD KNOW

- Unwrapped bakery goods may be contaminated with sesame seeds from other products, so only buy bakery products if they are pre-wrapped.
- Sesame seeds are often scattered about on delicatessen counters, so it is generally unsafe to buy from a delicatessen. Most delicatessen products are also available pre-packed, so you can buy these instead.
- 'Mixed spices' contain various spice seeds that may include sesame, so always check the ingredients label thoroughly.
- Most food manufacturers and supermarkets provide a 'free from sesame' list of their own-brand products (see Chapter 13, 'Eating In'). This will help you to choose suitable food to buy for a sesame-free diet.
- Sesame is used in some cosmetics. Since the passage of the Cosmetic Labelling Act in 1998, its inclusion must be listed among the ingredients.
- Sesame is sometimes used in medical preparations such as plasters, liniments, ointments and soaps. Always check the ingredients listings.
- Sesame oil may occasionally be present in medicines. Always ask your pharmacist to check any medication that you are planning to take.
- Sesame contains two natural antioxidants: sesamol and sesamoline. They both retain their properties during frying at high temperatures, which is why sesame oil is so highly prized by Chinese and Japanese chefs, who use it in many dishes. If you have a severe allergy to sesame, you should therefore avoid Chinese and Japanese cuisine.

Eating food that you have not prepared *yourself* carries the greatest risk of triggering a life-threatening anaphylactic reaction. This is partly because of the risks from cross-contamination (see Chapter 15) and partly because you might not recognise a dish as containing sesame if it is written in a language that is unfamiliar to you. Eating out requires a great deal of caution. The following are examples of foods that may lead to anaphylaxis because they include sesame:

- bread, biscuits and crackers,
- soups,
- mixed salads, salad dressings,
- vegetable burgers,
- sauces, marinades, stir-fry sauces,
- desserts,
- Chinese, Japanese, Greek, Mexican and Lebanese restaurant meals,
- humous, tahini and halva.

Humous is high on the list for triggering an allergic reaction, as are tahini and halva.

For more general advice on eating safely with a severe food allergy, see also Chapter 9 ('Food Labelling'), Chapter 13 ('Eating In') and Chapter 16 ('Eating Away from Home').

SHELLFISH-FREE AND FISH-FREE DIETS

As concerns about dietary fat and cholesterol have increased, seafood (shellfish) and fish (especially oily fish) have become a more prominent part of our diet. They can be eaten as a snack, sandwich filler, starter or main meal and are cooked in a variety of ways. Sushi, which is a raw fish delicacy, is also becoming very fashionable.

If you are allergic to one or more white or oily fish, it is generally suggested that, in the interests of safety, you should completely avoid all fish of that type.

SEAFOOD CLASSIFICATION

The scientific classification system for both plants and animals is divided into: kingdom, phylum, class, order, genus and species. Seafood is included in this classification, and a simple outline that includes the common names is given in the Table below.

Phylum	Class	Common name
Molluscs	Gastropods	Snail, abalone
	Bivalves	Clam, mussel, oyster
	Cephalopods	Octopus, scallop, squid
Arthropods	Crustacea	Crab, crayfish, lobster, prawn, shrimp
Chordates	Cartilaginous fish	Ray, shark
	Bony fish	Cod, salmon, tuna, etc.

See also Chapter 12 ('Cross-reactivity and Food Families').

Although all of these may give rise to food allergy, the *Crustacea* are the most common class of fish/seafood to cause this. Symptoms may include nausea, vomiting, diarrhoea, abdominal pain, rhinitis, rashes and, in extreme cases, anaphylaxis. Some people may get symptoms from just the smell and cooking vapours of shellfish and fish. If you are allergic to one or more members of a phylum, it is generally recommended that, in the interests of safety, you avoid all other members of that phylum.

Unlike some foods, cooking does not affect the allergenicity of members of the shellfish family.

'HIDDEN' SHELLFISH AND FISH

- **Ambergris**, which is obtained from the intestine of the sperm whale, is used in some perfumes.
- **Anchovy**, which is a small fish in the herring family, is often used as a flavour enhancer in Worcestershire sauce.
- **Aspic** is a savoury jelly, used as a glazing agent, that may be derived from fish.
- **Caviar** is the roe of the sturgeon and other fish; it may be used as a relish or garnish.

- **Chitin** is the organic base of the hard parts of crustaceans such as shrimps and crabs; it is used in hair conditioners, hair thickener, moisturising shampoos and skin care products.
- **Cod liver oil** is the oil extracted from the liver of the cod and related fish, and is often used as a nutritional supplement.
- **Isinglass** is a very pure form of gelatine that is obtained from the air bladders of some freshwater fishes, especially the sturgeon; it is used to clarify alcoholic drinks and jellies.
- **Sodium-5-inosinate**, prepared from fish waste, is used as a flavour enhancer.
- **Sperm oil** is found in the head of various species of whales, and is used for candle making.
- **Spermaceti wax** is a fatty substance found mainly in the head of the sperm whale and also in other whales and dolphins; it is used in medicines, candle making and cosmetics.
- **Squalene** is found in the liver of the shark; it is used in toiletries and cosmetics.
- **Vitamin D$_3$** (cholecalciferol) may be derived from fish oil, for use as a nutritional supplement.

Tales of the un*fish*spected

Fish and shellfish and their derivatives can sometimes be an ingredient of the following:

- artists' materials,
- beers and wines,
- cosmetics, toiletries, soaps (see also Chapter 9, 'Food Labelling'),
- glues and adhesives,
- nutritional supplements (e.g. vitamins),
- perfumes,
- pet foods, including fish food,
- washing-up liquids.

The list above is just for your information. Even if you are allergic to shellfish or fish, this does not mean that you will be allergic to these products. But if you are having a reaction and don't know why, one of these products might be the answer. Please discuss the matter with your allergy specialist.

To avoid fish and shellfish successfully, use products recommended by the Vegetarian Society and the Vegan Society. The Vegan Society lists suitable products in its handbook, *The Animal-Free Shopper* (see

Appendix 3 for details). To avoid the risk of cross-contamination, it would be wise for you to patronise vegetarian and vegan restaurants and guesthouses. This is especially important if the cooking vapours of shellfish or fish trigger your allergic symptoms.

WHEAT-FREE AND GLUTEN-FREE DIETS

Gluten is a protein found in wheat, rye, barley and oats. Ingredients to be avoided on food labels are these four grains, in all their various forms. Although oats do contain gluten, some people who are unable to tolerate gluten from other cereals are able to tolerate oats. Be sure to discuss with your doctor whether you can include oats in your diet.

WHAT IS THE DIFFERENCE BETWEEN WHEAT-FREE AND GLUTEN-FREE?

- **Wheat-free** means something that is free from wheat only.
- **Gluten-free** means something that is free from gluten – which can be found in barley, rye and oats as well as wheat. All of these *can* be eaten on a gluten-free diet if the gluten has been removed from them. The most common example of this is *de-glutenised wheat*: because the gluten has been removed, it is quite safe for it to be eaten on a gluten-free diet.

AVOIDING WHEAT

It is very difficult to avoid eating wheat, because:

- wheat is one of the staple foods of the British diet (e.g. bread, cakes, biscuits, pizza, pasta – the last usually made of durum wheat),
- wheat is present in a great many manufactured foods (e.g. flour as a thickener or 'filler' in soups and sauces, and sometimes even in curry powder).

You must scrutinise all food ingredients labels to make sure that you avoid wheat in all of its forms:

- all cereals of the *Triticum* species:
  - *Triticum spelta L* (spelt),
  - *Triticum poloncium L* (kamut),

- bran, wheat bran, wheat gluten, wheat germ,
- cereal filler, cereal binder, cereal protein,
- couscous,
- farina,
- flour, wholewheat flour, wheat flour, wheat starch,
- rusk,
- semolina, durum wheat semolina,
- starch, modified starch, hydrolysed starch, food starch, edible starch,
- vegetable protein, vegetable starch, vegetable gum,
- wheat, durum wheat.

Hydrolysed protein, hydrolysed vegetable protein and monosodium glutamate can be derived from wheat. However, the hydrolysis process breaks down the protein to a form that is unlikely to cause problems. So you should avoid these products only if you are extremely allergic to wheat – and, even then, discuss the matter first with your allergy specialist.

WHEAT SUBSTITUTES

If you can tolerate rye, oats, barley, corn and rice, you can eat baked products, cereals and pastas using these grains in place of wheat. In addition, unusual grains and flours such as amaranth, arrowroot, bean, buckwheat, lentil, millet, pea, potato, quinoa and soya, as well as groundnuts and seeds (e.g. pumpkin and sunflower), may be used in interesting combinations to make baked products and cereals. Many of the commercial wheat-free products are based on these ingredients. Less common and rather more difficult to cook with are sago and tapioca flours. Banana flour and chestnut flour are also available.

Cakes and biscuits made without wheat are rarely as successful as those with wheat, because they do not rise as well and often have an inferior texture. In recent years, though, specialist food manufacturers have made considerable improvements to the substitute commercial mixes and preparations. Many of these companies will send free samples of their products on request.

Wheat is contained in manufactured and processed foods where it is used for its versatile properties as a processing aid, a binder, a filler or as a carrier for flavourings and spices. Examples of items where wheat *may* be a 'hidden' ingredient include:

Artificial cream	Ketchup	Paté
Baked beans	Malt vinegar	Potato waffles
Canned meats	Meat pies	Processed cheese
Curry powder	Muesli	Sausages
Dry roasted nuts	Mustards	Scotch eggs
Fruit pie filling	Packet soups	Suet
Haggis		

Malt is a by-product of barley or other grains; therefore products containing this should be avoided.

You will find that many of the special products that are manufactured for gluten-free diets are made from de-glutenised wheat. Remember that these are *not* suitable if you are on a wheat-free diet.

AVOIDING GLUTEN

Coeliac disease and the skin condition dermatitis herpetiformis are the two main conditions that require strict adherence to a gluten-free diet. To help its members (and others) steer clear of food products that contain gluten, the Coeliac Society publishes *The Gluten-free Food & Drink Directory.* This is a small handbook (available in ordinary and in large print) containing a comprehensive list of manufactured products that are gluten-free. It is published annually and in between times there are regular updates about product changes. The handbook is available from the Coeliac Society, who also provides regular updates on its 24-hour phone hotline, on its website or by e-mail (see Appendix 1) or on BBC2 Ceefax during the first week of each month.

Gluten-free foods on prescription
A range of gluten-free products, including breads, pastas, biscuits, pizza bases and cake mixes are available on prescription at your GP's discretion. A full list of prescribable products can be obtained from your dietitian, from the Coeliac Society or from most pharmacist/chemist shops.

Substitute foods
Gluten-free substitutes usually supply approximately the same amount of vitamins and minerals as the foods they replace. They are prepared with special care, following good manufacturing practice

guidelines, to prevent contamination with ingredients that contain gluten. Quite a few of them are also free from other ingredients that can cause an allergic reaction in susceptible people, such as milk and egg. At the end of this chapter is a small selection of those that are available.

Top tips

- A full and regularly updated list of products available on prescription can be obtained from the Coeliac Society.
- Don't forget to ask manufacturers and supermarkets for their 'free from' lists. There are probably many foods stocked in supermarkets that will be suitable for your special diet but are not marketed as such.
- Most pharmacist/chemist shops have a list of wheat- and gluten-free products available (some on prescription and some to buy over the counter or by mail order).
- Contact the Coeliac Society if you require gluten-free communion wafers.
- Watch out for cross-contamination. It can easily occur with foods such as bread that are made up of crumbs, which seem to get everywhere. For example, if you share your butter with people who eat ordinary bread, you can pick up bread crumbs left behind by their knives! Ensure that your foods are stored and prepared away from those containing wheat and gluten (see Chapter 15, 'Cross-contamination').

LABELLING

Unfortunately, food labels do not tell consumers everything. Labelling will indicate the obvious presence of wheat or wheat flour but if the amount is less than 25% of a compound ingredient it can remain legally undeclared (see Chapter 9, 'Food Labelling'). Because of this, if you are allergic to wheat, you should consume only foods and products that are on a manufacturer's or supermarket's 'free from' list. If you are avoiding gluten, it is a good idea for you to obtain *The Gluten-free Food & Drink Directory* from the Coeliac Society; all the products in this handbook are free from gluten (at the time of going to press).

SPECIAL DIETARY PRODUCTS

Food type	Product details	Manufacturer
Baking and cooking	Gluten-free baking powder	Ultrapharm (Allergycare)
	Gluten-, wheat-, milk-, egg-free baking powder	Nutricia (Glutafin)
Biscuits	Lemon cookies free from gluten and wheat Roman cookies free from wheat	Doves Farm
	Apricot biscuits, chocolate cookies, ginger cookies, hazelnut cookies free from wheat and gluten	Gluten Free Foods (Glutano)
	Selection of biscuits free from wheat and gluten	Granny Ann (Itona)
	Selection of biscuits and cookies free from gluten	Lifestyle Healthcare
	Selection of biscuits free from wheat, gluten, milk and egg	Nutricia (Glutafin)
	Selection of biscuits free from gluten and wheat: Shortbreads: butter, pecan, lemon, swirls Cookies: carob hazelnut, ginger, peanut butter	Pamela's (Brewhurst)
	Selection of wheat- and gluten-free cookies and biscuits, including strawberry and chocolate rolls, low-fat varieties	Pleniday
	Selection of wheat- and gluten-free biscuits	SHS (Juvela)

Food type	Product details	Manufacturer
Bread and bread mix	Brown and white rice bread free from wheat, gluten, corn, egg, milk and soya	Gluten Free Foods (Barkat)
	White and brown rice bread, tapioca bread, maize bread – all free from wheat, gluten and dairy products	Ener-G
	Part-baked baguettes, rolls, bread mixes and sliced breads. Variety of products free from wheat, gluten, milk, egg, yeast and soya	Gluten Free Foods (Glutano)
	Sliced and unsliced, white, brown and high-fibre bread and rolls free from gluten	Lifestyle Healthcare
	Selection of speciality breads free from wheat and gluten: spicy onion, sunflower seed, sesame, etc.	Everfresh Natural Foods (Sunnyvale)
	Variety of bread, baguette and bread mixes free from wheat, gluten and egg	Nutricia (Glutafin and Rite-Diet)
	Selection of gluten-free bread and rolls	Pleniday
	Selection of gluten- and wheat-free breads, bread mixes, baguettes and croissants	Schär
Cakes	Gluten-free cakes: carrot and sultana, rich fruit, date and walnut, sticky ginger, cherry almond	Alternative Cakes
	Selection of cakes free from wheat and dairy products	De Rit
	Selection of cake and scone mixes free from wheat, gluten, egg and milk	General Dietary

Food type	Product details	Manufacturer
Cakes cont'd	Good selection of cakes free from gluten	Lifestyle Healthcare
	Dutch wheat- and egg-free fruit loaf	Mrs Crimble's
	Selection of cakes free from gluten: banana, date and walnut, lemon, fruit cake	Nutricia (Glutafin)
	Selection of gluten-free cakes: coconut rock cakes, fruit cake, madeleines, madeleines with raisins	Pleniday
	Selection of cakes free from wheat: carrot cake, gingerbread, fruit cake, Christmas cake	Village Bakery
Cereal bars	Selection of wheat-free cereal bars	Barbara's Bakery
Cereals	Gluten-free organic rice pops	Doves Farm
	Pure rice bran: free from wheat and gluten	Ener-G
	High-fibre soya bran	Granny Ann (Itona)
	Organic puffed rice cereal free from gluten and wheat	Kallo
	Muesli free from gluten and wheat	Pleniday
	Organic gluten-free quinoa flakes	Quinoa Real
Crackers	Wheat- and gluten-free maize crackers	Gluten Free Foods (Glutano)
	Organic rice cakes: sweet and savoury flavours	Kallo
	Crackers free from gluten, wheat, milk and egg	Nutricia (Glutafin)
	Variety of flavoured corn and rice crispbreads	Community Foods (Orgran)

Food type	Product details	Manufacturer
Flours	Rice flour, gram flour, gluten-free flour	Doves Farm
Gravy mix	Gluten-free gravy powder	Ultrapharm (Allergycare)
Noodles	100% rice noodles	Blue Dragon
	Brown rice noodles. Wheat-free noodles	Clearspring
Pasta	Big selection of gluten- and wheat-free pastas made from rice and soya. Many shapes and flavours	Community Foods (Orgran)
	Selection of gluten- and wheat-free pastas	Gluten Free Foods (Glutano)
	Gluten-free penne and fusilli	Lifestyle Healthcare
	Selection of gluten- and wheat-free pastas made from corn or rice	Mrs Leepers
	Selection of gluten- and wheat-free pastas	Pleniday
	Selection of gluten- and wheat-free pastas	Schär
Pizza bases	Gluten-free pizza base	Lifestyle Healthcare
	Gluten-free pre-cooked pizza base	Pleniday
Puddings and pastries	Selection of gluten-free pies, puddings, turnovers, Danish pastries and ready-to-roll sweet and savoury pastry	Lifestyle Healthcare
	White and brown pizza crust free from wheat, gluten, corn, milk, egg and soya	Gluten Free Foods (Barkat)
Snacks	Pretzels free from wheat and gluten	Gluten Free Foods (Glutano)
	Small selection of gluten-free savoury snack bars	Lifestyle Healthcare

Food type	Product details	Manufacturer
Stuffing and coating	Gluten-free herb and onion stuffing	Ultrapharm (Allergycare)
Vinegar	Organic brown rice vinegar	Clearspring

Many of these products are available on prescription (see Chapter 17, 'Help for People on Special Diets'). Your GP or pharmacist will be able to advise you on these products. Alternatively, contact the manufacturers direct (see Appendix 1).

SOYA-FREE DIET

Soya (also referred to as soy) is a legume from the food family *Leguminosae* (see Chapter 14, 'Cross-reactivity and Food Families'). It is a rare cause of anaphylaxis in the UK but when it does occur, complete avoidance of soya and its derivatives is necessary. This is more difficult than it sounds because in recent years it has become a major component of manufactured foods.

Examples of manufactured foods that may contain soya include:

Biscuits
Bread and bakery items
Cakes
Chinese food (contains soya sauce)
Cold delicatessen meats
Japanese food (contains miso)
Paté
Processed meats
Seasoned foods
Teriyaki sauce

The ingredients to avoid are:

Lecithin/Soya lecithin (E322)
Miso
Soy/Soya
Soya albumin
Soya bean sprouts
Soya beans
Soya flour
Soya milk
Soya nuts
Soya oil (especially cold-pressed)
Soya protein
Soya protein isolate
Soya sauce
Soya-based infant formula
Tempeh
Tofu
Vegetable protein, hydrolysed
Vegetable protein, textured

As well as the more obvious soya ingredients listed above, soya can be 'hidden' on an ingredients list as an *emulsifier, vegetable oil, vegetable stock, vegetable protein, vegetable starch* and *shortening,* so it is very difficult to choose soya-free foods with confidence. The safest way to buy soya-free foods is to obtain the 'free from soya' lists from supermarkets, food manufacturers and your dietitian (see also Chapter 13, 'Eating In'). With these, you can make sure that the food you purchase has no soya in it. Without them your diet will become very restricted indeed and probably nutritionally incomplete and unbalanced.

If it has not been confirmed that you are definitely severely allergic to soya, it is essential to check this with your allergy specialist. Otherwise, you may be following this very restrictive diet unnecessarily.

EATING OUT

If you are on a soya-free diet, eating out will probably be difficult unless dishes are made only from fresh ingredients. For ideas on how to eat out safely, see Chapters 14 ('Eating Away from Home') and 15 ('Cross-contamination').

TOILETRIES

Toiletries, perfumes and cosmetics containing soya or soya derivatives will be labelled according to the International Nomenclature of Cosmetic Ingredients (INCI). See Chapter 9 ('Food Labelling') for these names, which will enable you to identify them.

ALTERNATIVE FOODS

The following information should expand your diet, helping to make it more balanced. (If you are allergic to cow's milk as well as soya, this information will be particularly useful.)

Soya-free milks

Soya-free milks are generally based on oats, rice, coconut, peas or nuts.

Soya-free milks

Manufacturer	Product
Bart Spices	*Coconut* milk
Blue Dragon	Tinned *coconut* milk, fat-reduced *coconut* milk
Clearspring	Imagine: Rice Dream *rice* milk: original, vanilla, chocolate, carob, calcium-enriched. Range includes 1 litre and lunchbox size: original, chocolate, vanilla
Evernat	Organic *almond* drink, organic *hazelnut* drink
First Foods	Organic *rice* drink
Lima	*Rice* drink: original, vanilla, chocolate
Plamil	White Sun: *pea* protein alternative to milk: sweetened, non-sweetened
Provamel	*Rice* drink
Skane Dairy	Millmilk: *oat* drink: original, chocolate
Ultrapharm (Allergycare)	*Rice* milk powder
Vitariz	Organic *rice* drink

Alternatively, try making your own nut milks. Recipes for other home-made milks can be found in any vegan cookbook. (See Appendix 3 for a list of recipe books.)

Soya-free spreads
There is a good range of soya-free and dairy-free spreads, including supermarket own-brand varieties. The Table opposite lists soya-free spreads, and indicates the other ingredients that it is free from.

Other soya-free foods

'Cheeses'

- Oat-based soya- and dairy-free cream cheese, from First Foods.

Soya-free spreads

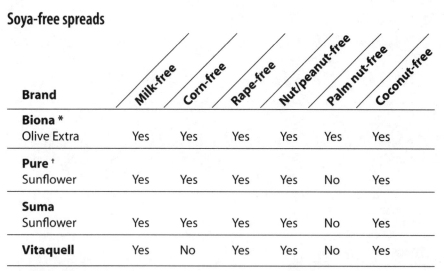

Brand	Milk-free	Corn-free	Rape-free	Nut/peanut-free	Palm nut-free	Coconut-free
Biona *						
Olive Extra	Yes	Yes	Yes	Yes	Yes	Yes
Pure †						
Sunflower	Yes	Yes	Yes	Yes	No	Yes
Suma						
Sunflower	Yes	Yes	Yes	Yes	No	Yes
Vitaquell	Yes	No	Yes	Yes	No	Yes

*Windmill Organics
† Matthews Foods

- Rice cheese slices, from Galaxy Foods. (Note, though, that they contain casein, which you should avoid if you are also allergic to cow's milk.)

Nutritional yeast-flakes
Engevita Nutritional Flakes, from Marigold Healthfoods, are available from most healthfood shops. (See this chapter's section 'Dairy-free diet' for details.)

Yoghurts and desserts
- Oat-based dairy-free and soya-free yoghurts, in various flavours, from First Foods.
- Yosa – soya- and dairy-free desserts, from NGT Associates. The flavours available are fruits of the forest, peach and passionfruit, pineapple, apple and banana – all with added calcium.
- Oat-based dairy-free 'ice-cream' in vanilla, strawberry or chocolate, from First Foods.

11
Allergy Prevention and Weaning

If you are planning an addition to your family, you will probably want to know how likely it is that the new baby might develop an allergy of some sort. You can then consider aspects of nutrition before conception, during pregnancy, during breast-feeding and when weaning the baby.

ATOPY

'Atopy' is the term for an inherited feature that makes it more likely that a person will develop an allergy. Not everyone who has atopy is necessarily going to develop an allergy but they are more likely to do so than someone without that tendency. Common allergic disorders include asthma, eczema, hay-fever and perennial rhinitis (like hay-fever but it lasts all year). The potential for someone inheriting an atopic condition is estimated as:

5–15% if neither parent is atopic
20–40% if one parent is atopic
40–60% if both parents are atopic
60–80% if both parents have the same atopy
25–35 % if one sibling (brother or sister) is atopic

A number of family studies have found that the mother's atopy is more likely than the father's to affect the next generation. This may be because the fetus is exposed to an allergic environment while in the womb.

Symptoms of an allergic condition may be triggered by various factors, related to the digestive tract, exercise, alcohol consumption, hormone levels, nutritional status and stress (see Chapter 4).

THE FATHER'S DIET

If you are planning for a baby with your partner, it is important to eat a varied balanced diet that fulfils all nutritional needs, for at least three months before conception. This is important for optimum healthy sperm production.

ADVICE FOR THE MOTHER

If you are trying for a baby, it is essential that your diet is varied yet balanced and meets all your nutritional requirements. You should also take folic acid supplements. Your dietitian can advise you on this and any other concerns you have.

Sometimes, if the mother- or father-to-be, their children, siblings or parents (first-degree relatives) are atopic, a pregnant woman may want to avoid the common 'allergy' foods during pregnancy: milk and milk products, eggs, fish and shellfish, and nuts.

If you are considering this, be sure to get expert advice from a dietitian. This is very important in helping you to make an informed choice and in ensuring that you take all the necessary replacement foods, so that your diet contains all the essential nutrients – both for you and for your baby. An 'exclusion diet' should only be undertaken under strict supervision by your dietitian.

Bottle or breast?

Breast-feeding has two major advantages for babies:

- it contains the mother's immunoglobulins,
- it is digested more easily.

This information is important for all mothers and their babies, but especially if the baby is from an atopic family.

Because food proteins such as lactoglobulin (from milk) and ovalbumin (from egg) can be found in breast milk, it is possible for a baby to have an allergic reaction to breast milk. If this occurs, it can manifest itself ('present') as a rash or diarrhoea. When the mother stops eating the relevant food, the baby's symptoms disappear. If your baby has been proven to have a food allergy and you are considering an exclusion diet, do get advice from a dietitian so that you can be sure of having a balanced and nutritious diet. Otherwise, your diet may become inadequate for you and your baby.

Unless your baby has had an allergic reaction to your breast milk, you should not stop breast-feeding. However, if you decide to do so and your baby is at high risk for developing allergies, you may be advised by your paediatrician to use a hypo-allergenic formula. For more information, see the section 'Formula milks for the allergic infant', below.

If you are already avoiding some foods in your diet for other reasons such as ethical, cultural or food preference, it is vital that your diet be assessed by a dietitian. The dietitian will give you the advice you need to obtain an adequate diet.

FORMULA MILKS FOR THE ALLERGIC INFANT

Infant formulas

Infant formulas are designed specifically to meet the nutritional needs of a growing infant. They comply fully with the UK regulations for infant formulas and are suitable for use as the sole source of nourishment for a young infant or as part of a mixed diet given to older infants and young children. A dietitian can help you make the correct choice of formula for your infant if you are in doubt.

The UK manufacturers of all infant products, including baby formulas, have removed nut and peanut derivatives from them to reduce the risk of early allergic sensitisation.

Soya protein formulas

Infant formulas based on soya are designed as a substitute for cow's milk formulas for babies who either have already developed an allergy or are at risk of doing so because of the family history. In the UK, government advice is that infants should be fed soya formula *only* if it is advised by a doctor.

Dental implications of soya infant formulas

Because soya infant formulas contain glucose syrups rather than lactose (which is the sugar occurring naturally in cow's milk), they are thought to have a greater potential to contribute to tooth decay (dental caries). It has been suggested that the way in which the soya formula is given is important if the development of dental caries is to be reduced. The longer the contact of the soya formula with the teeth, the greater the risk of tooth decay, so the baby's teeth should be brushed after each and every feed.

Soya phytoestrogens

Phytoestrogens are oestrogen-like substances that occur naturally in many plants and fungi (e.g. mushrooms). There is some concern that high levels of soya phytoestrogen could have an adverse effect on the hormonal development of infants. This is particularly the case in the USA where up to 25% of bottle-fed babies are now given soya formula rather than cow's milk formula. In the UK only 2% of bottle-fed babies are given soya formula.

Protein hydrolysate formulas

These are specifically designed for babies with an intolerance to milk. They contain cow's milk in which the proteins have been broken down by the process called hydrolysis, which makes them far less allergenic. These formulas are *not* suitable for infants who are known to have a severe allergy to cow's milk.

Amino acid formulas

Infants who cannot tolerate a protein hydrolysate can be given a formula made up of amino acids (the building blocks from which proteins are made). Amino acid formulas are sometimes called 'elemental formulas'. Because cow's milk is not used, this type of formula should not trigger an allergy.

Alternatives to cow's milk

It is essential to use a formula designed for infants. Soya milk, rice milk, oat milk, goat's milk and sheep's milk that are often used by older children and adults who are unable to tolerate, or choose not to take, cow's milk are not suitable for an infant because they do not contain adequate nutrition.

Goat's milk formula

In general, an infant who is allergic to cow's milk will often develop an allergy to goat's milk if this is used as a substitute. Therefore, goat's milk formula is not usually recommended as an alternative to cow's milk or cow's milk formula. There is some evidence that pea protein milk may be a suitable alternative

The Table overleaf shows whether the most popular infant formulas contain or are free from the three major allergens – soya, cow's milk and nut derivatives. (They are all egg-, wheat- and gluten-free.)

Type and indications	Product	Milk-free	Soya-free	Nut-free
Whey-dominant formulas. They are usually the first formula used	Cow & Gate Premium	No	No	Yes
	SMA Gold	No	Yes	Yes
	Farley's First	No	Yes	Yes
	Milupa Aptamil First (Cow & Gate)	No	Yes	Yes
	Boots Formula 1	No	No	Yes
Casein-dominant formulas marketed for hungry babies. Also suitable from birth	Cow & Gate Plus	No	No	Yes
	SMA White	Yes	Yes	Yes
	Farley's Second	No	Yes	Yes
	Milupa Milumil (Cow & Gate)	No	Yes	Yes
	Milupa Aptamil Extra (Cow & Gate)	No	Yes	Yes
	Boots Formula 2	No	No	Yes
Follow-on formula from 6 months of age. Contains higher levels of certain nutrients. *Not* for use in newborn babies	Cow & Gate Step-up	No	No	Yes
	SMA Progress	No	Yes	Yes
	Farley's Follow-on Formula	No	Yes	Yes
	Boots Follow-on Milk Ready to Feed	No	Yes	Yes
	Boots Follow-on Milk Powder	No	Yes	Yes
Soya-based. Used in lactose or milk protein intolerance	Cow & Gate Infasoy	Yes	No	Yes
	SMA Wysoy	Yes	No	Yes
	SMA LF (Lactose-free) Mead Johnson Enfamil Prosobee	No	No	Yes
	Farley's Soya Milk	Yes	No	Yes
Extensively hydrolysed formula for whole protein intolerance. No MCT oil	Mead Johnson Enfamil Nutramigen	No*	Yes	Yes
Extensively hydrolysed formula for multiple malabsorption. At least 50% MCT	Mead Johnson Enfamil Pregestimil	No*	Yes	Yes
	Cow & Gate Pepti-Junior	No*	No†	Yes

Type and indications	Product	Milk-free	Soya-free	Nut-free
Semi-elemental‡ formula based on soya and pork. No MCT	Milupa Prejomin (Cow & Gate)	Yes	No†	Yes
Elemental‡ formula	SHS Neocate	Yes	Yes	Yes

* Contains *hydrolysed whey* or *casein*, which may *not* be suitable if the infant has experienced an anaphylactic reaction but *is* suitable for any other cow's-milk-related allergy and intolerance.

† Contains *hydrolysed soya*, which is *not usually* suitable if the baby is at risk of a severe allergic reaction to soya but *is* suitable for less severe allergies and intolerances.

‡ An elemental formula is made up of protein, fat and carbohydrates in their simplest forms, with the addition of vitamins, minerals and trace elements.

MCT = medium-chain triglyceride(s) – one of the fat 'building blocks'

Note This Table is only a guide. *Always* read the product labels or check with the manufacturer if you are unsure about the contents of these or any other products.

WEANING

Once weaning is started, it is sensible to delay the introduction of foods that are commonly found to lead to allergies in children with a very strong family history of allergy: for example, eggs, wheat and gluten, soya, fish, shellfish, citrus fruits and nuts. The Table below suggests the earliest times that such foods should be introduced into the diet of an infant who might be at risk of developing a food allergy. For guidance on how long to delay, seek advice from the dietitian or paediatrician, who can help you make sure that the baby's diet is balanced and nutritious.

Peanuts and tree nuts should not be given to infants before they are three years old (see the section 'Peanut-free and nut-free diets' in Chapter 10).

Suitable weaning foods

Age	Weaning food	Comments
4 months	Baby rice	Make up with expressed breast milk, or a hypo-allergenic formula (e.g. Pregestimil/Pepti-Junior)
5–6 months	Pureed root vegetable (potato, carrot, swede, parsnip) Pureed fruit (banana, apple, pear)	Give singly or a combination of these
6 months	Cereals other than wheat Pureed meats (lamb or turkey, then pork or beef or chicken)	Give singly or a combination of these
8 months	Soya	
9 months	Wheat	Pasta, semolina, wheat-based breakfast cereal, bread
10 months	Fish	
11–12 months	Cow's milk (full fat)	Then yoghurt, cheese, butter, cream and other dairy products
1 year	Egg	Start in small amounts, well cooked (e.g. in cake), then boiled or scrambled eggs

All other foods may now be introduced except nuts and peanuts (and their products), which should not be given until the child is *at least* three years of age.

Weaning the infant with severe allergies

An infant who is at risk of having an anaphylactic reaction may need to be admitted into hospital when weaning foods are first introduced into the diet. This may be done, for example, if the infant has had an allergic reaction from just touching a food or if there has been a reaction when introducing other foods into the diet. The child's paediatrician will determine whether this is necessary.

Weaning foods for infants on special diets

Many of the companies that produce baby formulas also produce baby foods. These can be in powder form or in jars. The foods are well labelled as to their suitability for special diets. There is also a good amount of accompanying literature, including weaning charts, product information, recipes, nutrition information and ingredient listings. All meals are provided for – breakfast, lunch, supper – and include main courses and puddings.

For further information about what is available, contact the companies direct. The contact details are under 'Infant nutrition' in Appendix 1.

Peanut allergy

The Committee on Toxicity of Chemicals in Food, Consumer Products and the Environment (COT) was commissioned to look into the consumption of peanuts and peanut products by pregnant and breast-feeding women, infants and young children. They looked particularly at early exposure to peanut products and the risk of developing peanut allergy later in life. In June 1998 they reported the following:

- Atopy is an important factor in the development of peanut allergy.
- There is insufficient evidence available to give definite advice about not eating peanuts during pregnancy and breast-feeding or in early childhood.
- Advice, which is precautionary, recommends that:
  - women with allergic disease, or those with an allergic partner or child, may wish to avoid eating peanuts and peanut products during pregnancy and breast-feeding,
  - in common with the advice for all children, a susceptible baby should be breast-fed exclusively for the first four to six months,
  - during weaning, and until they are at least three years of age, infants should not be exposed to peanuts or peanut products.

Refined peanut oils should not contain peanut allergens. The use of products containing these oils in food, ointments or creams should not therefore result in an allergic reaction. In the extremely rare event of a reaction, it is most likely that it would be mild. If you are still worried, though, seek advice from an NHS allergy clinic. (See also 'Peanut-free and nut-free diets' in Chapter 10.)

Early weaning

Current medical advice suggests that all infants benefit from being breast-fed for at least four months. Solids should not be introduced into their diet until they are four months of age. Babies who are given foods other than milk in the first four months of life may have a higher risk of developing allergies later on. This is because babies' intestines, just like everything else about them, are still developing. While they are young the intestines are a bit leaky, allowing bits of protein and other substances directly into the blood stream. Once in the blood stream, these substances are exposed to the developing immune system. The substances are identified as foreign matter and the immune system starts producing antibodies against them.

However, many foodstuffs can pass through into breast milk in sufficient quantities to cause an allergic reaction. There is not yet enough information about the effects of dietary restrictions during pregnancy and breast-feeding to make it possible to advise women about a dietary strategy to prevent the development of allergy in their infants. For the present, therefore, it is best to eat a varied and balanced diet during pregnancy and while breast-feeding but to exclude very allergenic foods such as peanuts and shellfish if you have a family history of allergy.

RECIPE IDEAS USING FORMULA MILKS AND ALTERNATIVE MILKS

If your child is on a cow's-milk-free diet, the following examples of foods that can be made with formula milks or to which formula milk can be added will add variety to it. You may find them particularly useful if your child has difficulty taking enough milk alternative to meet nutritional requirements. It is recommended that all children under five years of age consume at least one pint (570ml/20 fl oz) of milk or milk alternative per day. Remember to use a formula designed for infants (as above) in children under a year old. Everyday soya, rice or oat milks are *not* suitable for them. If you are unsure about which milk substitute to use, ask your dietitian.

Savoury
These recipes should be bland, as infants do not need additional seasoning.

- basic white sauce
- creamed chicken
- fish pie
- french toast
- potato bake
- scrambled eggs
- shepherd's pie
- vegetable dinner

Desserts

- blancmange
- bread and butter pudding
- drinks
- fruit fool
- fruit trifle
- ice-cream
- jelly mousse
- milkshakes
- rice pudding

The manufacturers of formula milks usually have recipe booklets, available on request. Alternatively, ask your dietitian.

12
Cross-reactivity and Food Families

Cross-reactivity is defined as two or more allergens inducing similar reactions. The allergens may be from the same food group (related genetically) or from different food groups (not related genetically).

This chapter is for your information only. If you are having allergic reactions despite avoiding the food(s) you know you are allergic to, there may be an explanation. It may be that you are eating a food that is related – either genetically or chemically. But do *not* try to check this out on your own. Talk to your doctor, who will be able to do tests to look for an unknown or suspected allergy.

THE SAME FOOD GROUP

If you have an allergy to one food (e.g. fish or nuts), must you avoid other foods from the same food family (i.e. other fish or nuts)? There is no definite answer to this question. It is clear, though, that cross-reactivity in the same plant or animal family is uncommon, so it shouldn't be necessary for you to avoid all foods in a food family because you have an allergy to one of them. Leave them out of your diet only if you have had a reaction or if separate testing indicates that you should avoid them.

An exception to this advice is the crustaceans – for example, lobster, crab and shrimp. If you have an allergy to one shellfish, you must avoid them all. All bony fish have a protein called parvalbumin, which is know to provoke allergic reactions, so you should avoid all these fish. It is not known whether parvalbumin is found in cartilaginous fish such as shark, skate and dogfish. (Avoiding fish is discussed in Chapter 10 in the section 'Shellfish-free and fish-free diets'.) Animal milks (cow, sheep, goat) seem to have a high degree of cross-reactivity, as do eggs from different birds (chicken, duck, goose, turkey) and, to a lesser degree, tree nuts (Brazil nuts, walnuts, etc.).

DIFFERENT FOOD GROUPS

Scientific studies have revealed that some foods from unrelated groups nevertheless have common links in triggering an allergic reaction. Examples are listed below.

- Apple, carrot and celery
- Kiwi, poppy seeds, sesame seeds, hazelnut, rye
- Banana, avocado, kiwi, chestnut, fig, papaya, peanut, latex, soybean
- Apple, carrot, celery, potato, hazelnut, orange, tomato, peanut, birch pollen
- Banana, melon, ragweed
- Watermelon, ragweed pollen
- Apple, hazelnut, potato, birch pollen

If you have an allergy to one food in a group, you might well have a similar reaction to the others even though they belong to different food groups.

FOOD AND POLLEN

As you can see from the list above, cross-reactions can occur between inhaled pollen and food you eat. For example, if you are allergic to birch pollen, you could have an allergic reaction to celery. This is because they have similarities in their chemical structure.

TAXONOMIC GROUPS

The classification of organisms (taxonomy) outlined below may be useful in understanding cross-reactivity.

Taxonomic group	Comment
Species	A group of very similar individuals makes up a *species*
Genus (plural = genera)	Related species are grouped together in a *genus*. Related genera are sometimes grouped together in *tribes* and *sub-families*, which may themselves be grouped together in a *family*

Taxonomic group	Comment
Order	Related families are grouped together in an *order*
Class	Related orders are grouped together in a *class*
Phylum (plural = phyla)	Related classes are joined together in a *phylum*
Kingdom	Related phyla are joined together in a *kingdom* (e.g. the plant kingdom and the animal kingdom)

When cross-reactivity is discussed, it is usually in terms of food families. In practice, though, this is not necessarily the case, and all levels of the taxonomic classification should be considered.

Below are listed the various food families (with their Latin name in brackets). The main groups where cross-reaction is common are the cereals, shellfish, fish and tree nuts.

Plants

Banana family (*Musaceae*)
Bean and pea family
    (*Leguminosae*)
Bilberry family (*Ericaceae*)
Buckwheat family
    (*Polygonaceae*)
Cabbage family (*Criciferae*)
Carrot family (*Umbelliferae*)
Cashew family
    (*Anacardiaceae*)
Citrus family (*Rutaceae*)
Cucumber family
    (*Cucurbitaceae*)
Currant family
    (*Saxifragaceae*)
Daisy family (*Compositae*)
Fungi kingdom
Grape family (*Vitaceae*)
Grass family (*Gramineae*)
Mint family (*Labiatae*)
Mulberry family (*Moraceae*)
Onion family (*Liliaceae*)
Palm family (*Palmaceae*)
Potato family (*Solanaceae*)
Rose family (*Rosaceae*):
    Rosoideae; Prunoideae;
    Maloideae
Spinach family
    (*Chenopodiaceae*)
Walnut family (*Juglandaceae*)

Poultry and eggs

Duck family (*Anatidae*)

Grouse sub-family
  (*Tetraoninae*)

Pheasant sub-family
  (*Phasianinae*)

Pigeon family (*Columbidae*)

Snipe family (*Scolopacidae*)

Eggs

Fish and shellfish

Crustaceans (phylum *Crustacea*)

Fish

Molluscs (phylum *Mollusca*)

Meat and milk

Cattle family (*Bovidae*)

Deer family (*Cervidae*)

Pig family (*Suidae*)

Rabbit family (*Leporidae*)

13
Eating In

You could be forgiven for thinking that eating at home on a restricted diet is bland, boring and unimaginative. This is probably because it is all too easy to focus on the foods that you must avoid rather than those that are safe for you to eat. Unfortunately, the foods that you *can* eat never seem quite as appealing as those that you *can't*!

The information in this chapter will enable you to increase your food choices and add variety to your diet. Instead of feeling the odd one out at mealtimes, you will be able to share food and enjoy eating with your family.

HOW CAN I MAKE MY DIET MORE APPETISING?

Making food appetising both to you and to those you are catering for simply means cooking nutritious food that tastes and looks good. Although some recipes will need adapting by replacing certain ingredients with suitable alternatives, there will be many recipes that you can continue to use without making any changes. Experiment with new foods and special dietary products that are available, such as egg replacers or gluten-free items. And you can try out some new recipes, too.

Whether you want to prepare a snack, a gourmet dinner party or a birthday cake that everyone can eat, there are endless possibilities. There is plenty of scope for the reluctant cook, for those who love cooking and for those with a hectic lifestyle and no time to spend in the kitchen. You can continue to make use of fresh, dried, tinned, frozen and many convenience foods if you so desire.

Finding suitable foods and learning to make the most of what you can still eat are the key to an interesting and varied diet. It is easier than ever to achieve this now – many supermarkets now stock an increasing selection of 'special diet' foods, and healthfood shops and their range of products are becoming more abundant.

With good labelling, it is now possible to eat foods that were once avoided because they might have contained unsuitable ingredients. The labelling of manufactured foods has improved greatly over recent years, but on occasions it can be misleading. This may be because of the '25% rule' (see Chapter 9, 'Food Labelling') or because some consumers are ill-informed or lack understanding about food labelling. Another possible cause for misunderstanding is that the product originates in a country where food labels are less detailed. This can lead to your eating unintentionally an ingredient you are trying to avoid, so *beware*!

It is wise to consume only food you know is *definitely* free of the allergen that you are trying to avoid. There are several ways of identifying foods that are safe to eat, outlined below.

Labels indicating suitability for particular diets
Some foods specifically state on the label that they are suitable for a particular diet. For example, 'Suitable for a cow's-milk-free diet' or 'Nut-free'.

Supermarket 'free from' lists
Most supermarkets produce 'free from' lists. These are lists of all their own-brand foods that are free from a particular ingredient. If you have more than one food allergy, they will sometimes make up a list specifically for you; otherwise, you will need to check each list that relates to your allergies. 'Free from' lists are available free of charge and are updated regularly. (See Appendix 1 for contact details of the major supermarkets that provide this service.)

Always double-check the ingredients label on the product to ensure that it is still suitable for your particular diet. Ingredients sometimes change after the 'free from' list has been prepared – look out for 'New' or 'Improved' on the packaging. (For more information about food labelling, see Chapter 9.)

'Free from' lists via your dietitian
Only dietitians have access to 'free from' lists from the Food Intolerance Databank. This is an organisation that collates information on foods free from the major allergens. It obtains the information from food manufacturers who wish to participate. It is useful to obtain their 'free from' lists from your community or hospital dietitian in addition to the supermarket lists. (If you have not seen a dietitian and would like to do so, ask your doctor to refer you to one.)

Companies that, at the time of writing, participate with the Food Intolerance Databank are:

A G Barr Ltd
ASDA
Baxters of Speyside Ltd
Bernard Matthews Food Ltd
Best Foods (UK) Ltd
Birds Eye Walls Ltd
Bisto Foods Ltd
British Bakeries Ltd
British Sugar plc
Britvic Soft Drinks Ltd
Cadbury Ltd
Cereal Partners
Chivers Hartley Ltd
Copella Fruit Juices Ltd
Cow & Gate Nutricia Ltd
Dairy Crest Ltd
Doves Farm Foods
Eden Vale (Northern Foods)
Elsenham Quality Foods Ltd
G R Wright & Sons Ltd
General Dietary Ltd
HP Foods Ltd
J A Sharwood & Co. Ltd
John West Foods Ltd
Kellogg Supply Services
    (Europe) Ltd
Kitchen Range Foods Ltd
Kraft Jacobs Suchard Ltd
Larkhall Natural Health Ltd

Lofthouse of Fleetwood Ltd
Mars Confectionery
Matthews Foods plc
McDougalls Catering Foods Ltd
McDougalls Foods Ltd
Milupa Ltd
Morning Foods Ltd
Nestlé Rowntree
Nestlé UK Ltd
Nutricia Dietary Care Ltd
Pura Food Products Ltd
Quaker Oats Ltd
Rayner & Co Ltd
Scabrook Potato Crisp Ltd
SMA Nutrition
SmithKline Beecham Consumer
    Healthcare
St Ivel Ltd
Stratford-upon-Avon Foods
Tate and Lyle Sugars
Trebor Bassett Ltd
Vandemoortele (UK) Ltd
W & H Marriage & Sons Ltd
W Jordan (Cereals) Ltd
Walkers Nonsuch Ltd
Walkers Shortbread Ltd
Weetabix Ltd
Wrigley Company Ltd
Yakult Europe BV

Manufacturers' 'free from' lists

Many food manufacturers now produce their own 'free from' lists. This means that you can contact many of them direct to obtain a list of their products that are suitable for your particular diet. (See Appendix 1 for details of many of these well-known food manufacturers.)

Specialist food companies

Many specialised food companies produce foods and ingredients that can be used as alternatives to those you have to avoid on a restricted diet. (Appendix 1 lists many of these companies.) You will be amazed at the choice.

This area of the food industry has been expanding rapidly in recent years and is still gaining momentum. If you can spend some time finding out about and keeping up to date with 'special diet' products, your dietary horizons will blossom beyond your wildest dreams!

WHERE TO FIND OUT ABOUT 'SPECIAL DIET' PRODUCTS

- Chapter 10 and Appendix 1.
- Your dietitian.
- Your local allergy support group:
  - through the information and newsletters it provides,
  - by meeting and chatting with others who follow a special diet.
- Your local healthfood shop.
- By contacting and/or joining an association dedicated to food allergy (see Appendix 1).
- Your library.
- The Internet – there are various websites (see Appendix 2) that hold up-to-date information. (If you do not have access to the Internet, go to your local library who will either help you or be able to direct you to somewhere that can.)
- Your local pharmacist/chemist shop (choose a quiet time of day!).
- Your supermarket – take time to look thoroughly at what is available on the supermarket shelves, then discuss other possibilities with the manager.
- Health shows and fairs.

FINDING SUITABLE REPLACEMENT FOODS

Initially it will be trial and error to find replacement foods and ingredients that you like or are prepared to use. Some products may be unacceptable to you because of their taste, texture, price or availability. You may also have to cope with ingredients whose cooking properties are different from the products that they are replacing. Whatever the reason, do persevere. And keep trying new products developed for your particular allergy. For example, manufacturers of gluten-free products are constantly striving to produce gluten-free bread that tastes like the 'real thing' as well as expanding their range of other foods.

What about the cost?

Some companies will send you free samples of their products if you ask them, which is a good, cheap way to experiment with potential replacement foods. In some cases, they will keep your address on file and send you samples of new products they develop.

There are some state benefits and free prescriptions available for certain medical conditions, which can help with the cost of specialised products. This subject is discussed in Chapter 17.

What about my favourite recipes?

You can often continue to use your present recipes, replacing some ingredients as necessary. Be aware, though, that some recipes will need adapting. Some of these adapted recipes will be just the same or even an improvement on the original, while others will be a downright disaster. You just have to put this down to experience!

You can of course get cookery books specifically designed for special diets (see Appendix 3). They usually include a chapter on replacement ingredients. A bookshop will usually get these for you, or you can order them direct on the Internet if you prefer. Or your specific allergy support group may well have a recipe book.

Manufacturers of specialised food products usually provide a recipe book on request. All the recipes have been tried and tested, which is particularly useful for the novice.

Cookery courses

You may choose to go on a special-diet cookery course that will help to familiarise you with the use of replacement ingredients and give you lots of new recipe ideas. Courses on offer vary from one day to a year (see 'Special diet cookery courses' in Appendix 1).

Remember!

If you are working in the same area that has been used to prepare foods to which you are allergic, or using the same utensils, they must be thoroughly cleaned to prevent cross-contamination (see Chapter 15).

Plan meals enough in advance that you have all the required ingredients to make your chosen dish. This is especially important if some of the ingredients are not widely available.

Eating in successfully is really down to how much preparatory work you do and how you use the information you have about your particular allergy or allergies. Start with one or two simple dishes and before long your very own special recipes will have reached gourmet heights and those eating with you will look forward to trying your latest creation. Like anything new, adapting to your new diet will take time but, with perseverance, it will become routine.

The 'Eating In checklist' overleaf will help you remember the important points in the early days, and you might find it useful to look at it again from time to time.

By the time you have ticked all the boxes and spent a little time experimenting with recipes, your diet will no longer seem bland and unimaginative, and you will look forward with enthusiasm to the next innovation in your expanding recipe book.

MY EATING IN CHECKLIST

☐ I have seen a dietitian.

☐ I have obtained a Food Intolerance Databank 'free from' list from the dietitian.

☐ I understand food labelling.

☐ I understand the 25% rule.

☐ I have a 'free from' list from all my local supermarkets and know how to use them.

☐ I have contacted food manufacturers for their 'free from' lists.

☐ I always double-check food labels when using 'free from' lists.

☐ I have obtained samples of replacement ingredients for special food products where they are available.

☐ I have tried replacement ingredients and foods.

☐ I have tried out lots of new recipes.

☐ I have joined an allergy support group.

☐ I have joined appropriate support organisations and receive regular newsletters from them.

☐ I have visited the library, bookshop or Internet websites for more information.

☐ I have checked with my GP or dietitian for information on any foods available on prescription for my allergy.

☐ I plan meals well in advance, especially if I know that I am going to be busy or if I am cooking for others.

☐ I always clean utensils and work-surfaces before I start preparing food.

☐ I have tried more than one type of replacement food rather than giving up on replacement foods because I didn't like the first couple that I tried.

14
Eating Away from Home

When you are on a restricted diet, eating away from home can be difficult. This may be due to the practicalities involved or because of other people's attitudes, ignorance and misunderstandings.

There is usually a way round most difficulties but it can sometimes be tedious and take away the pleasure of eating out. This chapter will help you to deal with issues that may occur in everyday situations so that you will be able to eat away from home safely and confidently.

'Eating out' encompasses many different settings, including the following:

- barbecue
- bed and breakfast
- Brownies/Cubs/Scouts
- buffet
- church
- cinema
- conference
- course
- dance
- dinner party
- fair or fête
- health club
- hospital
- hotel
- nursery
- party
- picnic
- pub
- restaurant
- sandwich bar
- school or school outing
- shopping trip
- take-away
- theatre

- tourist attractions
- travel
- university or college
- wedding

You will have to make specific arrangements that will vary according to where you are going and what you are doing, but below are some basic guidelines that you should always follow if the experience is to be as hassle-free and as safe as possible.

BASIC GUIDELINES FOR EATING OUT

- Understand your food allergy, and be able to answer questions about it competently and clearly when asked by those preparing food for you.
- Always contact, in advance, the person who is catering for you to tell them about your special diet. Clear written guidelines are ideal in minimising the risk of ambiguity and they can be kept for future reference. The person doing the catering – whether a friend, a colleague or a professional caterer – will then know that they are well prepared and be confident that the food they are providing is suitable.
- Try to persuade the caterer that making food for all members of the party in accordance with your diet will probably make life a lot easier for them as well as safer for you.
- Find out answers to questions you are unsure of before eating anything you may be allergic to.
- Do *not* under any circumstances eat any food prepared by someone else *unless you are sure* it is definitely safe for you.
- Check the ingredients of any manufactured foods used by the chef to ensure that they are all suitable.
- Have the confidence to say what is required to ensure that the food you consume is safe for you. If the caterer is unable or unwilling to provide what you need, suggest that you bring your own.
- Take your own food if it has been agreed with the person who usually does the catering. You can make this less conspicuous by:
  – making sure the person doing the catering and arranging the event knows in advance that you are doing this,

- ensuring that your food looks the same as everyone else's by finding out in advance what the others will be eating and obtaining (e.g. borrowing from a restaurant) similar crockery so that yours doesn't look out of place,
- taking your food earlier in the day to wherever you will be eating (cover it to prevent cross-contamination) and explain any issues both verbally and in writing to save time and trouble later when staff are often busy and perhaps less receptive,
- or taking your food to the kitchen when you arrive at the function so that it can be served to you at the same time as the rest of your party. (Make sure that those serving are aware of the cross-contamination issues (see Chapter 15).)

- Don't avoid situations because they will involve eating; instead, plan well ahead so that food no longer becomes an issue.
- Speak to the chef direct rather than via the waiting staff, who will not necessarily relay your needs to the chef correctly.
- Take your own special ingredients, pans and utensils for the chef to use and any seasoning that will enhance the enjoyment of your food. (But give them plenty of notice!)
- Patronise the same restaurant/pub/eating house again if you have had a successful eating experience. It is better to return on a quieter day at a quieter time of day if possible (8 p.m. on a Saturday night with no forewarning is not a good time to ask for a special meal!).
- Be aware that food allergens can appear in the most unusual ways – so check:
  - communion wafers (they usually contain gluten),
  - home-made jams (they often contain butter – used to clarify the 'scum' during making),
  - mulled wine and cocktails (they could contain anything, and the fruit might have been cut on a board with allergens on it),
  - the sugar bowl (this almost certainly contains globules of milk).

If you are at risk of having an anaphylactic reaction:

- DO *carry your adrenaline at all times*.
- DO understand when to use adrenaline and be prepared to use it. (See Chapter 5, 'Your Anaphylaxis Contingency Plan'.)

Taking your own food

Remember that many establishments *will* allow you to take food that you have prepared yourself, and they will heat it up for you if required. If the food is covered in cling film, you can be sure it will be completely safe, which means you can concentrate on enjoying yourself instead of worrying and the staff can relax!

SPECIAL OCCASIONS

If you are organising an important function such as a wedding, christening or anniversary, you will probably want to employ a caterer to prepare the food. Caterers can be unhelpful or ignorant about food allergy but do not give up! There *are* caterers out there who are experienced in this aspect of food preparation and will be willing to cater for your special function. It is wise to plan the catering well ahead so that you have plenty of time to find someone you are happy with and trust to do exactly as you request. I am living proof of this: at my own wedding I had a completely dairy-free spread of delicious food.

GOING INTO HOSPITAL

You may, at some time in your life, have to go into hospital. This may be for a planned operation or it might be unexpected because you have been involved in an accident.

Whatever the case, you need to be aware that even hospitals are not always as informed as they should be about food allergies. My editor has coeliac disease and, a few years ago, was in hospital for nearly two weeks because she broke her leg quite badly. Although her dietitian was based in that hospital, she discovered that the kitchen didn't really understand what a 'gluten-free diet' entailed. One evening, all she got for supper was three scoops of mashed potato, even though there were items on the menu that would have been perfectly acceptable for her!

Someone else I know has a severe allergy to milk and dairy products. When she went into hospital to have her baby, she decided not to risk the unnecessary complication of an anaphylactic reaction from hospital food, and got her mother to bring in *all* her food. This might seem extreme but, if you have a severe food allergy, it is better to be safe than sorry.

SEVERE FOOD ALLERGY

Eating away from home can be a problem if you have a severe food allergy. The risk seems to be greater in some establishments, depending on the range of food to which you are allergic. The following is an example of these risks for someone with an allergy to peanut/nut and their derivatives. The risk can be greater in Oriental restaurants because:

- Foods often contain more ingredients.
- Nuts and peanuts tend to be used more than in Western-style cooking.
- Ingredients may be 'hidden' within a dish and therefore are not recognised.
- A strong-flavoured dish can mask the taste of the individual ingredients (including any nuts).
- A spicy food can mask the initial sensation of an allergic reaction.
- Language problems may hinder understanding between the person with the allergy and the restaurant staff.
- Nut and peanut allergy is rare in Oriental countries, which can result in a poor understanding of the problem in Oriental establishments.

In a joint effort by the Ministry of Agriculture, Fisheries and Food (MAFF), the Anaphylaxis Campaign and representatives from the food industry, a guidance document and pack about anaphylaxis and food allergy awareness has been produced. It has been designed specifically to help the catering industry understand the issues and to strive to provide suitable foods for people with a food allergy. The pack consists of a booklet, posters and stickers, and is available from Admail 6000 (see Appendix 1 for details.)

15
Cross-contamination

'Cross-contamination' is what happens when allergens are transferred from one food or food ingredient to another. In a very few instances this may result in a previously safe food becoming unsafe. If you have a severe food allergy and eat this food, thinking it is safe, you may well develop an allergic reaction. This chapter considers some of the issues.

Cross-contamination is a significant issue, but unfortunately not one that is understood by many of the general, non-allergic, community. It can happen in a wide range of circumstances, but occurs most commonly during food manufacturing and food preparation. Another type of cross-contamination occurs when food allergens are transferred not to another food but to an object or person. The list given in the section 'Out and about' is included because it may explain why, for example, you always get an itchy face after using a phone you share with a colleague.

FOOD MANUFACTURE

Food manufacturers are now much more aware of food allergy and the importance of labelling their products clearly. This is discussed in Chapter 9. They are also improving their manufacturing practices to prevent accidental cross-contamination.

FOOD PREPARATION

This includes food prepared at home – over which you probably have at least some control – and food prepared elsewhere.

Shopping
Many aspects of shopping can lead to cross-contamination. For example:

- Delicatessen bags may have been handled by assistants touching foods that you are allergic to.

- Food obtained from a bakery or delicatessen, because foods are not wrapped.
- Food handlers' hands may be contaminated with an allergen and then used to touch your food.
- Handling other people's food to which you are allergic. The food may even be on the outside of an unopened packet because another packet has split and spilled its contents.
- Supermarket conveyor belts may have had food allergens spilt on them and not been cleaned thoroughly.

In the kitchen
Look out particularly for the following.

- Utensils and work surfaces that are not thoroughly clean (e.g. a grater that has cheese stuck in it and you are allergic to cheese).
- Odd-shaped containers that are hard to get thoroughly clean.
- Ovens with burnt on food which then falls onto your food.
- Cooking oil that has been used for frying many different food items, including some to which you are allergic.
- Flour or other packets having been handled by someone whose hands are contaminated with a food to which you are allergic.
- Spillages in the fridge: food to which you are allergic may spill onto your food. (For example, milk kept on the top shelf could cause an anaphylactic reaction if it spilt onto the food of someone severely allergic to milk.)
- Used spoons and knives put back in a sugar bowl, marmalade jar, butter dish or coffee jar.
- Inadequate washing of ingredients (e.g. a tomato from a self-service container might have been handled by others).
- Inadequate handwashing before and between food preparation.

Eating
The main risks of cross-contamination when you are eating arise from:

- Drinking from someone else's cup.
- Using someone else's cutlery.
- Eating a normally safe food that has been placed by food that is unsafe for you (e.g. eating grapes from a dish that also contains cheese if you are allergic to cheese).

It is essential that caterers preparing food for someone with a severe allergy understand the issues of cross-contamination. Unless you advise them about this, they probably won't realise that only a minute quantity of an allergenic food will trigger a life-threatening reaction. Never assume that a catering establishment will know about all the issues regarding food allergies. Your specific needs should be clearly written down and talked through with the person who will be preparing and serving your food.

The Anaphylaxis Campaign has produced a factsheet entitled *Severe Food Allergies: Guidance for Caterers.* It includes information for caterers, guidance for serving staff and specific points for all staff. The factsheet contains some general points that apply to the preparation and serving of foods for all severe food allergies and specific 'nut-aware' advice. If you know of a caterer or catering establishment that does not have a copy, do tell them about it, as they would probably welcome its guidance. Alternatively, you can make up your own guide based on this factsheet, but including ideas from your own experience.

OUT AND ABOUT

Be aware that things you come into contact with in general living may trigger an allergic reaction if they have been touched by someone who has been in contact with a food to which you are allergic. For example, you might develop a very uncomfortable, itchy skin rash if you touch 'contaminated':

- door handles,
- pens and pencils,
- telephones,
- fridge doors,
- teaspoons used to stir drinks,
- trays previously used to carry food or drinks,
- washing-up cloths, washing-up brush, tea-towels and towels.

You may have only a mild reaction or just a rash, or perhaps no reaction at all. But it helps to be aware of the possibilities!

PERSONAL CONTACT

You might easily react with an itchy rash in the following circumstances or contacts.

- Expressed breast milk, if the mother consumes food to which you are allergic.
- Kissing, especially on the lips or cheeks.
- Pet foods, which can be transferred onto pets' fur if they lick themselves and you then stroke or cuddle them.
- Shaking hands.
- Vomit, if the baby or person has consumed anything that contains food that is unsafe for you.

I am sure you can think of many many more, especially those that are pertinent to *your* allergy.

A good way to ensure that you don't inadvertently expose yourself to the possibility of cross-contamination is to have a checklist. You may find the one given here helpful, and perhaps you can add to it.

MY CHECKLIST TO PREVENT CROSS-CONTAMINATION

- ☐ I always use gloves when I go anywhere near food to which I am allergic.
- ☐ I always wash fresh fruit, salad and vegetables before eating them.
- ☐ I never drink from a cup/glass or use cutlery/crockery unless it has been thoroughly washed.
- ☐ I never kiss someone without making sure that they haven't recently eaten the foods that I am allergic to.
- ☐ I never eat (suitable) foods from a buffet unless I can take mine first.
- ☐ I always inform anyone catering for me about the risk of cross-contamination, giving them plenty of notice.
- ☐ I always offer to take my own food to social events or make myself available to help during preparation when others are nervous about catering for my needs.
- ☐ I never risk eating anything that I suspect may be contaminated with food that is unsafe for me.
- ☐ I always carry my medication and action plan for treatment, just in case cross-contamination occurs.

Enjoying Life

16
Holidays and Travelling

Getting away from it all is an important part of life. We all need a break from our routine, and benefit from the rest, relaxation and recharging the spirit, as well as a bit of indulgence, too! This chapter tells you about options that are available to you when deciding on a holiday, whether in the UK or abroad. The information will also be useful if you are travelling on business.

TRAVELLING OR HOLIDAYING IN THE UK

Much of Chapter 14 ('Eating Away from Home') applies when you are travelling in the UK or staying somewhere on holiday.

Bed and breakfast (B&B) and guest houses

Vegan guest houses are usually automatically free of egg, fish, shellfish, meat and milk. (Vegetarian guest houses will not usually be egg- and milk-free.) If you have a milk or egg allergy, it will generally be completely safe to go to a 100% vegan guest house. Do be aware, though, that some vegan establishments have eggs and cow's milk available for their non-vegan guests. It may still be safe to stay there if these foods are kept separately, with no risk of cross-contamination.

For details of places to stay and eat, consult:

- Appendix 1, section 'Accommodation and eating out'.
- Action Against Allergy (contact details in Appendix 1), who will provide a list on request.
- British Allergy Foundation (details in Appendix 1), who have a Holiday Accommodation List.
- Coeliac Society (details in Appendix 1), who have a list of accommodation and holiday places to stay where the proprietors or a member of the family are coeliac and they are used to cooking gluten- and wheat-free food. Many of them are also happy to cater for other special diets.
- Vegan Society (details in Appendix 1).
- 'Eating out and holiday accommodation' section in Appendix 3.

When you find a place where you feel confident, tell the Anaphylaxis Campaign, the British Allergy Foundation and Action Against Allergy about it, so that others can enjoy the facilities with confidence, too. And, of course, use it again yourself!

TRAVELLING OR HOLIDAYING ABROAD

You might think that it is impossible to eat safely and confidently when you are away from your own kitchen and in a foreign country but this is not so. If you take on board the following advice, you will minimise the risks.

It is, of course, essential to be fully prepared. You can do this by reducing the risks and thus prevent an allergic reaction, but also planning what to do if there is an emergency. If you need a referral to an allergy specialist in European countries outside the UK, you should seek a doctor who is a member of the European Academy of Allergy and Clinical Immunology.

Reducing the risk to prevent an allergic reaction
Well in advance of your holiday, obtain a set of translation cards that explain your allergy in the language of any country that you are travelling through or to. You can buy these from the British Allergy Foundation, provided you give them at least one month's notice. Some specific allergy support groups (e.g. the Coeliac Society) can also provide this sort of information.

I strongly recommend that you also obtain a letter from your GP stating that you are carrying medication and why. Show the letter to customs officials if there are any queries, which should prevent the possibility of your medication causing problems or being seized by them.

Travelling by air, sea or channel tunnel
If you are travelling by aeroplane or any other mode of transport where food is provided, it is often possible to order a special meal (e.g. milk-free, nut-free, wheat-free). *Beware*, though, as these meals may not be what they claim, and eating them could have serious consequences if you cannot get to medical care quickly. It is often easier and safer to take food that you have prepared yourself for these journeys.

If you are travelling in a group, make sure that all members of your party know about your allergy. If you are travelling alone, be sure to carry identification that will warn others of your allergy in the event that you are unable to tell them. In either case, also tell a member of the crew about your allergy.

Carry all medication in your hand luggage for easy accessibility. Do not place it in a bag that could get lost or mislaid.

If you are travelling by aeroplane and are allergic to nuts, phone the airline and request a nut-free flight. Many airlines now have a specific policy for nut-free travel. Some people have reported that they have suffered an allergic reaction while travelling on an aircraft. The cause is thought to be the free peanut snacks distributed to all passengers from the beverages trolley. When the packets are opened, the peanut dust gets into the air and is circulated and recirculated around the aircraft cabin. The Anaphylaxis Campaign has contacted a number of airlines to ask if they are willing to remove the peanut snacks from a flight if adequate notice is given; many say they will. For a list of the airlines agreeing to do this, contact the Anaphylaxis Campaign (details in Appendix 1).

Arriving at your destination
As soon as you reach your destination, find out how to use the telephone so you are prepared if an emergency arises. Learning how to call a doctor and an ambulance are your priorities. Alternatively, take your mobile phone so that you have access to immediate telephone contact. (Make sure that you can use it abroad!) If you decide to take your mobile phone, it would be a good idea to programme the local 'emergency' numbers into it at the start of your holiday. They include the hospital, the doctor, a taxi company, your holiday rep (if you have one) and the proprietor or manager of your accommodation.

Find out where the nearest hospital is. It may be useful to contact the hospital at the beginning of the holiday to tell them where you are staying and what your requirements might be. Then, if an emergency does occur, all parties are well informed. You may be happier to find a hospital that has a comparable standard of healthcare to the UK.

Accommodation
If you are at risk of a very severe reaction, it is probably wise to choose accommodation where you are in control of the food preparation. Choose either self-catering accommodation, so that you can prepare your own food, or catered accommodation where you are completely confident that the chef understands and is prepared to cater for your special needs.

Self-catering is the probably the best option, because you are completely in control of the food that you are eating. With a kitchen of your own you can explore local markets and enjoy all the local fresh produce. However, a major part of a holiday is often the welcome escape from the domestic chores, so self-catering may not appeal to you. (If you are abroad on business, you may not have time to do marketing and cooking!) However, many hotels now have rooms with basic kitchen facilities. Using these, you can prepare your own meals but still dine with others who are eating the hotel food. They can enjoy not having to cook while knowing that you can all enjoy eating together without worrying about your allergy.

You may prefer to choose a holiday with a representative (holiday rep) who has a good living and working knowledge of the country you are visiting. It would be advisable to make sure they have written details of your medical condition and any action plan that you have formulated. Take their mobile phone number if they have one so that they can be contacted without delay if the need arises.

Food issues on holiday

Choose a holiday destination where the locals and you can understand one another and where food labelling regulations and allergy awareness are comparable to the UK. You can find this information by contacting the embassy of the country to which you are travelling or by calling the MAFF information line (see Appendix 1).

Avoid any situations that have triggered an allergic reaction in the past. And never eat or drink anything unless you are completely confident that it is safe to do so.

Preparing food yourself

- Take your own food that you have prepared to your destination. Do not risk taking any new foods that you have not tried before.
- Ensure that all utensils in your self-catering apartment are scrupulously clean. This includes the fridge, cooker and grill pan.
- On arrival, check that the cooker hob and oven are working satisfactorily. If they are not, you may wish to change rooms or put in a request for them to be fixed as a matter of urgency.
- Take advantage of fresh foods from the local markets. Perhaps you could try to make some dishes similar to those at the local

restaurants so that you don't feel left out. (See also Chapter 13, 'Eating In'.)

- Always take your own food on days out so that you are not tempted to eat food that may not be safe for you.

Food prepared by others

If you do decide to eat out, make sure that you take translations and always check ingredients and preparation methods if they are not made clear on the menu. Always speak to the chef direct rather than via the waiter. If the chef is too busy to speak to you, he is probably too busy to take on board what you are trying to tell him so it is advisable to go elsewhere.

Most holidays involve alcohol, perhaps including the occasional cocktail. If you are having a cocktail, make sure that the shaker has been thoroughly washed, as otherwise it may contain traces of allergen. Even better – choose something else, such as a glass of wine or a bottled or canned soft drink.

Avoid drinks that have fruit added, because the boards and knives may be contaminated with food allergens. Think carefully before you have ice cubes. Although it is rare that they are the cause of an allergic reaction, it *is* possible. Those from an ice-making machine are more likely to be safe than those made in a fridge.

If you are allowing someone else to cater for you, always double-check and confirm in writing that you both have the same understanding of your requirements and that they will be able to meet your special needs. Take a copy of the letter with you on your holiday, in case they renege on their promises. (See also Chapter 14, 'Eating Away from Home'.)

PLANNING FOR AN EMERGENCY

- Make sure that you have adequate medication in case you need it for self-administration. Not doing so could have fatal consequences. Carry this medication at all times as well as ID and an action plan on the preferred procedure for administration. This will be especially important if you are unable to administer it yourself. (See also Chapter 5, 'Your Anaphylaxis Contingency Plan'.)
- Carry an action plan in case of emergencies. Try role-playing this to ensure that everyone who might be involved understands

what to do and is confident to implement the plan swiftly and efficiently in an emergency. You may wish to get medical help when writing the action plan or have it checked over when you have written it – ask your GP or your doctor at the allergy clinic.

- Make sure that the action plan can be located immediately by all members of your party and that they know how use it.
- You must locate the nearest hospital and know how to get there quickly if you need treatment. To speed up the treatment, you should have details of the nature of your allergy and the action required if you have a serious reaction. If you are going abroad, make sure that you have clear translations.
- Obtain adequate travel insurance. It is essential that you tell the sales assistant about your allergy and ensure it is documented on the application form; otherwise, you may not be covered if you make a claim.
- If you are travelling through or to European Union countries, obtain form E111 – available from the post office. When stamped at the post office, it allows free reciprocal healthcare. Remember to carry it with your other travel documents.
- If you are worried that your medication will deteriorate because you are going to a country with a hot climate, you may wish to purchase a small cooler in which to keep it. One such cooler is the FRIO-PACK which is available from FRIO UK (address in Appendix 1). The FRIO Wallet will keep your medication at constantly low temperatures. It requires no refrigeration and is very simply and quickly reactivated by water. It can be used time and time again. Many others are available via the Internet, mainly from the USA.
- Carry spare copies of your guidance notes with you to hand to chefs (have them laminated so that they can be cleaned easily if they get splashed in a busy kitchen).
- You may find it useful to take this book with you as a reference guide, especially if others you are travelling with are not used to your allergy. Two other books that you may find useful are the *Travellers Guide to Health*, which is a Department of Health publication, and *Allergies at your fingertips* (see Appendix 3).

As well as all the above points, make sure you read – or re-read – Chapter 14 ('Eating Away from Home').

OTHER ISSUES

Taking new medication and going to the dentist when you are abroad are two scenarios to talk through with your NHS allergy specialist before you go. Do not agree to use any new medication or injections while abroad unless you are sure it is safe for you to do so.

SUMMARY

Below is a checklist for you to work through to make sure that you have done everything possible to ensure a relaxed and safe holiday.

CHECKLIST FOR TRAVELLING

☐ I have asked my doctor:
  – for a brief medical history to take with me,
  – to help me formulate or check my action plan for emergency use.

☐ I have obtained a translation describing my allergy and my emergency action plan and have extra copies to give to key people.

☐ I have obtained the name, address and phone number of a doctor at my holiday destination.

☐ I have obtained the name, address and phone number of the hospital nearest to where I will be staying.

☐ I have obtained the emergency phone number of the country I'm going to (e.g. 999 in the UK).

☐ I have arranged adequate medical holiday insurance, advising the insurer about my allergy.

☐ I have noted my National Insurance number and obtained my E111 from the post office.

☐ I have obtained an extra supply of my medication.

☐ I have packed my health insurance details.

☐ I have taken a copy of all the documents listed above, and will carry a set with me at all times on holiday and leave another in my room.

☐ I have a list of people at home who should be contacted in the event of an emergency.

17
Help for People on Special Diets

Having to use 'special diet' foods and other allergen-free products can be expensive. They usually cost more than ordinary food and ingredients. This chapter outlines some ways that may help you financially or just with useful advice.

FREE PRESCRIPTIONS

Even if you are not entitled to free prescriptions for the medication you need for an allergy, it may be useful to know the criteria to qualify for this in case your circumstances change.

You are entitled to exemption from prescription charges if you:

- are a permanent resident in a nursing/residential home (at least partly funded by the local authority),
- are a war-disabled pensioner,
- are aged 60 or over,
- have a child under the age of one year,
- are on a low income (holding certificate HC2),
- are receiving Income Support,
- are pregnant,
- are under 16, or under 19 and in full-time education,
- have:
  - a continuing disability,
  - a permanent fistula requiring continuous surgical dressing or appliance,
  - diabetes insipidus or other hypopituitarism,
  - diabetes mellitus and are taking medication for it,
  - epilepsy requiring continuous anti-convulsive therapy,
  - a form of hypoadrenalism (including Addison's disease),
  - hypoparathyroidism,
  - myasthenia gravis,
  - myxoedema.

In addition, people receiving the following state benefits are automatically entitled to free prescriptions:

- income-based JobSeekers Allowance,
- Family Credit,
- Disabled Person's Tax Credit.

Other people in receipt of means-tested benefits may also be eligible. If you think that you might be eligible, consult leaflet HC11 – *Are You Entitled to Help with Health Costs?* – available at main post offices and Benefits Agency (DSS) offices and from many GP surgeries and pharmacy/chemist shops.

People who are exempt from paying prescription charges are now asked to provide proof of their exemption when they collect their prescription. Failure to do so may mean that they have to pay the prescription charge.

PREPAYMENT CERTIFICATE ('SEASON TICKET') FOR PRESCRIPTIONS

If you need lots of prescriptions, it may save money in the long run to pre-pay the prescription charges with a prepayment certificate, often called a season ticket. This can be purchased for a period of four months or one year. Once the initial fee has been paid, all prescription charges will be free for the chosen period. If you are likely to need six or more items in four months or 15 or more in a year, it is probably worth your while getting a 'season ticket'. Further information about them is available from most pharmacy/chemist shops, GP surgeries and post office counters (ask for form FP95).

OVER-THE-COUNTER MEDICINES

Many medicines on prescription are also available over the counter – without a prescription – direct from the pharmacy/chemist shop or pharmacy department in the supermarket. Sometimes the cost will be less than the prescription charge. To ensure that you are getting medicines in the most economical way, it is useful to check this out with the pharmacist.

NON-COW'S MILK FORMULA ON PRESCRIPTION

Babies who are unable to tolerate cow's milk formula are entitled to get an alternative on prescription from the GP. Because babies are exempt from paying prescription charges, this will be free.

GLUTEN-FREE PRODUCTS

Many gluten-free products (basic food items such as bread, flour and pasta) are prescribable by the GP for people with coeliac disease. Occasionally, GPs agree to prescribe these products for someone with another food allergy or intolerance. This is more likely to happen if the person has seen a dietitian or been to an allergy clinic where a formal diagnosis has been made.

WHOLE-EGG REPLACER

Whole-egg replacer is available on prescription. It can be used as a replacement for eggs in recipes, adding variety to the diet. (See also 'Egg-free diet' in Chapter 10 for suggestions for replacing the properties of whole egg and egg white that you can buy or make from everyday ingredients.)

STATE BENEFITS

Social Fund
This is a state benefit that is usually accessed in relation to a special need. For example, if a washing machine or vacuum cleaner is required to keep your house dust-mite-free for a child with severe eczema, or an oven is required to cook special dietary products in, this fund may pay for it. Details can be obtained from your local Benefits Agency office.

Disability Living Allowance (DLA), care component
This is available for anyone under 65 who needs extra personal care in the long term. For example, the extra care for a child with eczema who requires time-consuming treatments such as wet wraps or for the extra time that is required to shop and cook for a special diet. The care part of the DLA has three rates, depending on the amount of care the person needs.

Invalid Care Allowance

If someone is receiving DLA at the upper or middle rate, their main carer may be entitled to claim Invalid Care Allowance if they are providing at least 35 hours of care.

Claiming state benefits

To claim any of the above benefits, first get the relevant leaflets from your local Benefits Agency office (the phone number will be in your telephone directory).

If your claim is unsuccessful, you can then appeal against the decision. To do this you will require medical reports from your GP and hospital consultant. Advice from the local Citizens Advice Bureau (CAB) may also be useful in preparing your case.

NON-FINANCIAL SOURCES OF HELP WHEN ON A SPECIAL DIET

There are many ways to find help and advice about special diets. They include:

- Action Against Allergy,
- allergy specialist,
- allergy support group,
- Anaphylaxis Campaign,
- Baby Milk Action,
- British Allergy Foundation,
- British Alternative Milk Advisory Service,
- dietitian,
- district nurse,
- food manufacturers,
- GP,
- health fairs/shows,
- health visitor,
- healthfood shops,
- internet websites,
- library,
- paediatric nurse,
- special diet cookbooks,
- supermarkets,
- Vegan Society.

And many many more – add your own sources below so that you can refer to it in times of need. (Contact details of the organisations listed above can be found in Appendix 1.)

18
Career and Leisure Choices

Depending on the nature of your food allergy and any other allergies that you may have, it would probably be useful to consider issues that could affect your choices of career and hobbies. It is sensible to look at this factor before you start training for a career in one of these areas.

FOOD ALLERGY

If you have a severe food allergy, the following careers may prove to be unsuitable choices:

- bakery,
- chef/catering staff,
- childcare/nanny
- cocktail bar worker,
- food factory,
- food handler,
- food shop worker,
- kitchen hand,
- waiter/waitress.

OTHER ALLERGY

Many people with severe food allergies often also have asthma, eczema or hay-fever. In view of this, it would be useful to bear this in mind when planning to invest time and finances in career and leisure choices. The following are examples of careers that may need extra thought beforehand:

- carpenter,
- carpet seller,
- cement worker,
- cleaner,

- factory worker (some),
- florist,
- hairdresser,
- jockey,
- nurse,
- pub worker,
- vet/veterinary nurse,
- waiter/waitress,
- washer-upper.

OTHER CHOICES

Don't worry if the lists seem rather long. It is not that these careers are totally unsuitable, just that you may experience difficulties and would need to find alternative ways of doing some things.

Here are some preferable career choices:

- administrator,
- artist,
- author,
- dancer,
- designer,
- doctor (except if you have a latex allergy),
- engineer,
- journalist,
- lawyer,
- lecturer,
- newsreader,
- police officer,
- receptionist,
- salesperson,
- secretary,
- teacher,

etc., etc., etc.!

LEISURE

There are certain leisure activities that might be unsuitable if you have a severe food allergy or are allergic to grass, pollen, animal fur, dust and other allergens. It is useful to make your leisure choices with this in mind. Think about the relevant choices and try them out. Whatever you do, though, *enjoy yourself and have some fun*!

There is absolutely no reason why you cannot enjoy a fulfilling work and social life because of your severe food allergy, or any other allergy. Being informed and understanding your allergy and knowing what action to take if a severe reaction is triggered are the key to successfully putting it to the back of your mind and getting on with the things that matter to you in life.

Glossary

Terms in *italic* in the definitions are also given in the Glossary

acute short term, intense; the opposite of *chronic*

adrenaline adrenaline (also called epinephrine) is a hormone produced by the adrenal glands when we exercise or are feeling afraid or stressed. It acts on the blood vessels (arteries and veins) to maintain normal blood pressure and circulation. In *anaphylaxis* it is given as an emergency injection to do just this, to reverse the symptoms of the reaction

allergen a substance – protein molecule (e.g. nut protein, milk protein, egg protein) – that can trigger the body's *immune system* to produce *antibodies* and thereby cause an *allergic reaction*. (See also *antigen*)

allergic reaction an immune reaction involving a specific type of *antibody* – immunoglobulin E (IgE)

allergic rhinitis *inflammation* of the lining of the nose, caused by an *allergic reaction*

allergy an abnormal or inappropriate reaction of the body's *immune system* to a substance (an *allergen*) that would normally be harmless

anaphylactic shock/anaphylaxis a sudden, severe *allergic reaction* to an *allergen* that can be life-threatening; if untreated, it can lead to dizziness, shortness of breath, wheezing, palpitations, a serious drop in blood pressure and collapse

angio-oedema presence of fluid in the deep layers of the skin (the dermis), particularly of the face, eyes, lips, tongue and throat, as a result of an *allergic reaction*

antibodies produced by the *immune system* in response to a foreign substance, antibodies circulate in the blood serum and help to fight infection and foreign elements called *antigens*. (See also *immunoglobulins*)

antigen a substance capable of inducing an immune response. (See also *allergen*)

antihistamines drugs that block the action of *histamine*

Arachis hypogaea the botanical name for the peanut plant

arachis oil peanut oil

asthma a *chronic* lung disease in which *inflammation* of the airways and twitchiness of the airway wall muscles make it difficult to move air in and out of the lungs, and causes the symptoms of wheezing, coughing and tightness of the chest, making it difficult to breathe

atopic/atopy an inherited tendency to develop an *allergy* or allergies such as *asthma*, *eczema* and hay-fever

bronchi the branching airways leading to the lungs

challenge test a test that involves a substance (e.g. a suspect food) being given in increasing amounts to see if an *allergic reaction* will occur, and, if so, at what level of exposure

chronic persisting for a long time; the opposite of *acute*

circulatory collapse the blood vessels in the tissues (the capillaries) dilate and become more leaky. Because of this, less blood returns to the heart to be pumped round the body, blood pressure falls and oxygen delivery to the tissues becomes less efficient. Eventually, oxygen delivery is so poor and the blood pressure is so low that the circulatory system collapses and so does the person

complementary therapies non-medical treatments that may be used in addition to conventional medicine. Popular examples are acupuncture, aromatherapy, homoeopathy and osteopathy

conjunctivitis *inflammation* of the conjunctiva, which is a delicate membrane that lines the eyelids and covers the eyeballs; it causes itchy, watering red eyes and is often associated with *allergic rhinitis*

COT Committee on Toxicity of Chemicals in Foods, Consumer Products and the Environment: a committee of independent experts that advises the Government

corticosteroids a group of chemicals produced naturally in the body by the adrenal glands, and are vital for the body's defences against infection and stress. They can also be manufactured (and are often called 'steroids'). Used as anti-inflammatory drugs they suppress the body's *immune system* and thereby dampen the inflammatory over-reaction. They come as creams, inhalants, tablets and eye drops

cross-reactivity associations between allergies due to common *allergens*. For example, some people who are allergic to latex get symptoms from eating banana, avocado or kiwi fruit

crude oil unrefined oil that may contain sufficient quantities of protein to induce an *allergic reaction*

desensitisation see *immunotherapy*

dietitian a professional with medical training in using diet as a therapy for illness and who gives advice about all aspects of food and diet

eczema a *chronic* inflammatory condition of the skin that makes it itchy. In mild cases the skin is dry and scaly but it can become red, blistered and weepy if severe

epinephrine see *adrenaline*

exacerbate make worse

food allergy the adverse health that results from a specific immune response

food and symptom diary a diary in which you list all the food and drinks you have consumed and any symptoms experienced during a set period

gluten a protein found in wheat, barley, oats and rye

ground nut a member of the *Leguminosae* family that grows in the ground (e.g. peanut). Other members of this family include peas, beans and lentils

histamine a chemical released by the body during an *allergic reaction*. Histamine causes *inflammation* and the symptoms of *allergy*.

hives another name for *urticaria*

hydrocortisone see *corticosteroids*

immune system the body's mechanism of resistance to external factors, thereby protecting itself. In allergic people the *immune system* over-reacts to agents that are harmless to non-allergic people

immunoglobulin E (IgE) an *antibody* (one of five classes of human immunoglobulin) that is involved in *allergy* and *anaphylaxis*

immunotherapy gradually increasing doses of an *allergen* are administered until an allergic person can tolerate exposure without developing major symptoms. Also called 'desensitisation'

incidence the number of new cases of a disease that occur during a particular time in a defined population

inflammation swelling and redness; in an *allergic reaction* the purpose of inflammation is to set up a chain of chemical actions that dilute and destroy the *allergen* that triggered the response

intolerance when the body reacts inappropriately – but without producing *immunoglobulin E* (IgE) – to a particular substance. Examples are lactose intolerance and irritable bowel disease (IBS)

lactose a sugar found only in animal milks (including human milk). It is most commonly referred to as the sugar in cow's milk

Leguminosae the pea and bean (legume) family of foods, of which the peanut and soya bean are part

mast cells cells containing *histamine*, which is released during an *allergic reaction*

mucosa the mucus membrane that lines many parts of the body, such as the gut and the airways

nettle rash another name for *urticaria*

open challenge a test for food allergy in which both the doctor doing the testing and the person being tested know what foods are being given

osteoporosis weak brittle bones

pareve a category of kosher food: it contains neither meat nor dairy products, nor their derivatives, and it is not processed on equipment that has processed products containing meat

patch test a skin test for diagnosing which *allergens* someone is allergic to; it is particularly useful for contact *eczema*, or dermatitis

prevalence a measure of the number of people in the population with a particular medical condition at any one time. For example, if we say that the current prevalence of severe food allergy is 2%, we mean that 2% of the population currently has a severe food allergy

prophylactic something given as a protective or preventative measure

protocol a formal written plan setting out the action to be taken in a certain situation

provocation test see *challenge test*

rash a skin eruption

RAST (radio-allergosorbent test) a diagnostic blood test for detecting *immunoglobulin E* (IgE) *antibodies* produced by your *immune system* against a suspected *allergen*

rhinitis inflammation of the lining of the nose. The symptoms include a blocked nose, runny nose and sneezing

skin-prick test a diagnostic test used to identify which *allergens* someone is allergic to. Pricking gently through a drop of *allergen* extract placed on the arm may produce a small swelling after 10–15 minutes, which indicates the presence of an *allergy*. The procedure is painless, gives rapid results and is probably the most commonly used and most informative allergy test

tree nut a nut that grows on a tree (e.g. Brazil nut, hazelnut, macadamia nut, pecan, walnut, almond)

urticaria a skin ailment characterised by a rash with *weals*, resembling nettle rash. Also called 'hives' or 'nettle rash'

weal a bump or ridge of skin

ABBREVIATIONS

AAA Action Against allergy
AAIA Asthma Allergy Information Association
AFAD Association for Allergic Disorders
BAF British Allergy Foundation
BNF British Nutrition Foundation
BSACI British Society of Allergy and Clinical Immunology
CAB Citizens Advice Bureau
COT Committee on Toxicity of Chemicals in Foods, Consumer Products and the Environment
DfEE Department for Education and Employment
DOH Department of Health
FAC Food Advisory Committee
FSA Food Standards Agency
INCI International Nomenclature of Cosmetic Ingredients
MAFF Ministry of Agriculture, Fisheries and Foods
NICE National Institute of Clinical Excellence
SCOPA Seed Crushers and Oil Producers Association
SPT skin-prick test

Appendix 1
Useful Addresses

USEFUL ORGANISATIONS

Action Against Allergy
PO Box 278
Twickenham
Middx TW1 4QQ
Tel: 020 8892 2711
Fax: 020 8892 4950
A support charity, providing
information (including holiday and
accommodation), suppliers list,
newsletter advice on specialist
referrals. Send s.a.e. for information.

Admail 6000
London SW1A 2XX
Tel: 08459 556 000 (MAFF
Publications)
Fax: 020 8694 8776
Websites: www.maff.gov.uk;
www.foodstandards.gov.uk
Distributes information on severe
food allergies, on request, to the
catering industry. Please quote the
following codes for the products
required: poster: PB3317; booklet:
PB3318; stickers: PB3406 and
PB3407.

AFAD (Association for Allergic Disorders)
24 Chiltern Road
Ramsbottom, Bury
Lancs BL0 9LF
Tel: 01706 828 256
Founded in 1993 by Christine Barker
to link people with allergies and
parents of children with allergies, to
share information and experiences.
Monthly newsheet. Specialist packs
on specific allergies and recipes for
special diets. Small membership fee.

Allerayde Ltd
41 Barton Road
Bletchley
Milton Keynes MK2 3HU
Tel: 01636 613 609
Fax: 01636 370 762
Website: www.allerayde.co.uk
Manufacturer and distributor of
adrenaline pens: Adult Anapen,
Junior Anapen and Anapen Trainer.
Also produces a training video and
booklet about anaphylaxis and use of
the Anapens, which is especially
useful for schools and for use in
hospital clinics.

Allergy Asthma Information Association (AAIA)
Box 100
Toronto
Ontario M9W 5K9
Canada
Tel: (416) 679 9521/1-800 611 7011
Fax: (416) 679 9524
Websites: www.aaia.ca
www.cadvision.com/allergy
Canada-based organisation, also called Calgary Allergy Network, dedicated to helping people with allergy and their families, and to promote allergy awareness and knowledge. Newsletters; 'No peanuts/nuts please' poster; allergy buttons ('Don't feed me . . . I'm allergic'); pen and puffer kit (small carry-bag for the EpiPen and asthma puffers) and EpiPen replacement plastic tubes.

ALK-ABELLÓ (UK)
2 Tealgate
Hungerford
Berks RG17 0YT
Tel: 01488 686 016
Fax: 01488 685 423
Website: www.ALK_ABELLO.com
Imports and distributes the Epipen, EpiPen Junior and EpiPen Trainer in the UK. The trainer pen can be purchased directly from them for around £5.00.

Anaphylaxis Campaign
PO Box 275
Farnborough
Hants GU14 6SX
Tel: 01252 542 029
Fax: 01252 377 140
Website: www.anaphylaxis.org.uk
Set up in 1994 to spread awareness and information about life-threatening allergic reactions. By mid-2000 there were 6,000 members across the UK, most being the parents of children with peanut/nut allergy. The Campaign produces a range of educational news sheets and videos. It has an extensive support group network.

Baby Milk Action
23 St Andrews Street
Cambridge CB2 3AX
Tel: 01223 464 420
Fax: 01223 464 417
Website: www.babymilkaction.org
Produces and distributes information and resources on infant nutrition.

British Allergy Foundation
Deepdene House
30 Bellegrove Road
Welling
Kent DA16 3PY
Tel: 020 8303 8525
Helpline: 020 8303 8583
Fax: 020 8303 8792
Website: www.allergyfoundation.com
Booklets, leaflets, quarterly newsletter, support group network, translation cards for travel abroad. A helpline for advice and information. A modest annual subscription.

British Alternative Milk Advisory Service
A service that sets out the historical, nutritional and ethical backgrounds. It is run by Plamil Foods, which see.

British Dietetic Association
5th floor, Elizabeth House
Suffolk Street
Queensway
Birmingham B1 1LS
Tel: 0121 616 4900
Fax: 0121 616 4901
Website: www.bda.uk.com
National association to which most dietitians belong. Distributes the 'free from' lists produced by the Food Intolerance Databank. Has produced a guidance sheet for dietitians on peanut allergy.

British Goat Society
34–36 Fore Street
Bovey Tracey
Newton Abbott
Devon TQ13 9AD
Tel: 01626 833 168
Provides details and literature on goat's milk and products.

British Nutrition Foundation
High Holborn House
52–54 High Holborn
London WC1V 6RQ
Tel: 020 7404 6504
Fax: 020 7404 6747
Website: www.nutrition.org.uk
Provides information on nutrition in the UK.

British Society for Allergy and Clinical Immunology (BSACI)
66 Weston Park
Thames Ditton
Surrey KT7 0HL
Tel: 020 8398 9240
Fax: 020 8398 2766
Website: www.soton.ac.uk/~bsaci
Aims to improve allergy services. Produces an annually updated list of NHS allergy clinics in the UK.

Coeliac Society
PO Box 220
High Wycombe
Bucks HP11 2HY
Tel: 01494 437 278
Hotline: 01494 473 510
Fax: 01494 474 349
Website: www.coeliac.co.uk
e-mail: foodlist@coeliac.co.uk
A registered charity that produces and distributes useful and informative literature on living with the coeliac condition, including a quarterly newsletter called *The Crossed Grain*, a list of products available on prescription and an annual directory listing gluten-free manufactured foods. Regular updates to the directory can be obtained from their 24-hour phone hotline, by e-mail or from their website (updated monthly) or on BBC2 Ceefax during the first week of each month.

Cosmetic, Toiletries & Perfumeries Association (CTPA)
Josaron House
5–7 John Princes Street
London W1G 0JN
Tel: 020 7491 8891
Fax: 020 7493 8061
Website: www.ctpa.org.uk
Information on the INCI names of cosmetic ingredients, and about suitable cosmetics, perfumes and toiletries, depending on your allergy and what you are trying to avoid. Note that they deal only with enquiries from professionals.

Davies Engraving
48 Norton Road
Walsall WS3 4AX
Tel/Fax: 01922 693 722
Makers of individual plastic badges that can be used as an allergy ID badge. Variety of shapes (animals, clowns, etc.) and colours for children.

Department of Health (DoH)
Richmond House
79 Whitehall
London SW1A 2NF
Tel: 020 7210 4850
Freephone 0800 555 777 (health literature line)
Fax: 020 7210 5661 (Public Enquiry Office)
Website: www.doh.gov.uk
Produces and distributes literature about public health, including matters relating to food allergy.

DfEE Publications
PO Box 5050
Sherwood Park
Annesley
Notts NG15 0DJ
Tel: 0845 60 222 60
Fax: 0845 60 333 60
Website: www.dfee.gov.uk
Department for Education and Employment. Publisher of *Supporting Pupils with Medical Needs: A good practice guide*, which is very useful for the management of anaphylaxis in schools.

Food Allergy Network (FAN)
10400 Eaton Place
Suite 107
Fairfax VA
22030-2208 USA
Website: www.foodallergy.org
A non-profit-making US organisation devoted to educating the public about food allergy. Publishes six newsletters a year and offers an excellent range of other resources that can be purchased by mail order.

Food and Chemical Allergy Association
27 Ferringham Lane
Ferring-by-Sea
Worthing BN12 5NB
Information on allergy-induced illness, particularly with food, chemicals and environmental pollution. Will refer enquirers as appropriate to other associations and doctors in this field.

Food Commission
94 White Lion Street
London N1 9PF
Tel: 020 7837 2250
Fax: 020 7837 1141
Website: www.foodcomm.org.uk
A national non-profit-making
organisation campaigning for safer,
healthier food. Supporters receive the
Food Magazine.

Food and Drink Federation (FDF)
6 Catherine Street
London WC2B 5JJ
Tel: 020 7420 7143
Fax: 020 7379 8538
Website: www.fdf.org.uk
Produces annually updated *Food
Allergen Advice Notes* and deals with
current food issues for food
manufacturers.

Food Intolerance Databank
Leatherhead Food RA
Randalls Road
Leatherhead
Surrey KT22 7RY
Tel: 01372 376 761/822 374
Websites: www.lfra.co.uk
Produces information on suitable
foods for diets free from: dairy, wheat,
soya, egg, BHA, BHT, sulphur
dioxide, benzoate and azo colours.
Information available only through a
dietitian.

Food Standards Agency
Room 6121, Hannibal House
PO Box 30080
London SE1 6YA
Tel: 0845 757 3012
Fax: 020 7972 2340
e-mail: Consumer@info.maff.gov.uk
Website: www.foodstandards.gov.uk
Sets standards in relation to food
issues and ensures that these are
being kept to by food producers,
distributors and caterers. At the
same address is the Food labelling
and Standards Division.

Frio UK Ltd
PO Box 10
Haverfordwest SA62 5YG
Tel: 01437 741 700
Fax: 01437 741 781
Website: www.friouk.com
Manufacturer and distributor of the
FRIO-PACK, designed to keep the
EpiPen and Anapen or other
medication at a constant
temperature. Particularly useful
when travelling in a hot country.

Golden Key
1 Hare Street
Sheerness
Kent ME12 1AH
Tel: 01795 663 403
Fax: 01795 661 356
Website: www.goldenkeyuk.co
Provides engraving service for SOS
identification bracelets, necklets, key
rings, badges. Very competitive
prices. Individual service by mail
order.

Latex Allergy Support Group
PO Box 27
Filey YO14 9YH
Tel: 07071 225 837
Members receive the quarterly
newsletter, fact sheets and list of
everyday items that contain latex
and those that are latex-free. Annual
membership £10. Information and
advice available on request.

**MAFF (Ministry of Agriculture Fisheries
and Food)**
Nobel House
17 Smith Square
London SW1P 3JR
Tel: 0645 556000 (to order
publications)
Helpline: 0345 573 012 (for queries)
Website: www.maff.gov.uk
For general enquiries concerning
food policy and legislation.

Medic-Alert Foundation
1 Bridge Wharf
156 Caledonian Road
London N1 9UU
Tel: 020 7833 3034
Freephone: 0800 581 420
Fax: 020 7713 5653
Website: www.medic-alert.co.uk
Produces a selection of identification
'jewellery' with an internationally
recognised medical symbol and 24-
hour emergency telephone number,
for people with hidden medical
conditions.

Medi-Tag
37 Northampton Street
Hockley
Birmingham B18 6DU
Tel: 0121 200 1616
Fax: 0121 212 3737
Website: www.medi-tag.co.uk
Produces identification jewellery,
including a selection of pendants,
bracelets and watches.

Merton Books
PO Box 279
Twickenham
Middx TW1 4XQ
Tel: 020 8892 4949
Fax: 020 8892 4950
Website: www.merton-books.co.uk
Publishers and stockists of a large
selection of books on allergies by
mail order. Allergy book list also
available from Action Against
Allergy (which see).

**Midlands Asthma and Allergy Research
Association (MAARA)**
12 Vernon Street
Derby DE1 1FT
Tel: 01332 362 461
Fax: 01332 362 462
Websites: www.maara.org/
www.usersglobalnet.co.uk/~aair/
anaphylaxis.htm
A research and support association
offering advice and information for
people with allergies and their
families. *Research (AAIR)* is the
Leicester branch of MAARA (with its
own website).

National Asthma Campaign
Providence House
Providence Place
London N1 0NT
Tel: 020 7226 2260
Helpline: 0845 01 02 03
Fax: 020 7704 0740
Website: www.asthma.org.uk
Advice and useful booklets on
asthma. Its helpline is staffed by a
team of specialist asthma nurses.

National Eczema Society
Hill House
Highgate Hill
London N19 5NA
Tel: 020 7281 3553
Helpline: 0870 241 3604
Fax: 020 7281 6395
Website: www.eczema.org/
Provides information leaflets, a
newsletter and a helpline for people
with eczema and for parents of
children with eczema. A support
network covers all areas of the UK.

National Osteoporosis Society
PO Box 10
Radstock
Bath BA3 3YB
Tel: 01761 471 771
Helpline: 01761 472 721
Fax: 01761 471 104
Website: www.NOS.org.uk
Information regarding osteoporosis,
its prevention and treatment, with a
network of local support groups.

SOS Talisman
Talman Ltd
21 Grays Corner
Ley Street
Ilford
Essex IG2 7RQ
Tel: 020 8554 5579
Fax: 020 8554 1090
Website:
www.sostalisman.btinternet.com
Produces a selection of identification
jewellery available by mail order and
through branches of Boots.

UCB Institute of Allergy
UCB House
3 George Street
Watford
Herts WD18 0UH
Tel: 01923 211 811
Fax: 01923 229 002
Website:www.
TheUCBInstituteofAllergy.ucb.be
Information and action, by research
and advice, and informing both
health professionals and the public
on pertinent issues.

Vegan Society
Donald Watson House
7 Battle Road
St Leonards-on-Sea
East Sussex TN37 7AA
Tel: 01424 427 393
Fax: 01424 717 064
Website: www.vegansociety.com
Has an excellent selection of vegan
cookery books and travel guides.
Distributor for Condomi Condoms
(milk-protein-free condoms). The
website is an excellent source about
foods and products free from milk,
eggs, animals, fish and shellfish.

Vegetarian Guides Ltd
PO Box 2284
London W1A 5UH
Tel: 020 7580 8458
Fax: 0870 121 4721
Website:
www.vegetarianguides.co.uk
Guides to vegetarian and vegan
restaurants, cafés, B&Bs, hotels, bars,
etc., in cities and countryside around
the world. Especially useful for
anyone avoiding, meat, fish, eggs,
milk and dairy products.

MANUFACTURERS AND SUPPLIERS OF SPECIAL DIET PRODUCTS

Where no contact address or
telephone number is given, ask your
local healthfood shop for details of
the product. Alternatively, contact a
distributor direct (such as Brewhurst
or Goodness Foods, listed in the next
section).

Alpro UK Ltd
see Vandermoortele (UK) Ltd

Alternatives – Specialist Bakers
Unit 8c
Northumberland
NE65 0PE
Tel: 01665 712 360
Website: www.
altcakes.free-online.co.uk
Selection of homemade cakes free
from eggs and dairy (vegan): carrot
and sultana; cherry almond; coffee
walnut; choc chip; rich fruit; sticky
ginger; banana and apricot; date and
walnut; lemon Madeira. Gluten-free
white or brown breads. Buy direct by
mail order or through a healthfood
store on request or via distributor
Brewhurst.

Amy's Kitchen
c/o Windmill Organics [distributor]
Selection of pot pies, pizzas, ready
meals, Asian meals, burritos,
burgers, snacks and desserts – many
of which are dairy-free, egg-free and
vegan.

Animal Aid
The Old Chapel
Bradford Street
Tonbridge
Kent TN9 1AW
Tel: 01732 364 546
Fax: 01732 366 533
Website: www.animalaid.org.uk
Organisation selling vegan wines,
bars and boxes of dairy-free
chocolates and fudge.

Annie's Naturals
c/o Marigold Health Foods
[distributor]
Website: www.anniesnaturals.com
Organic salad dressings and
vinaigrettes, each suitable for a
variety of special dietary
requirements: gluten-free, vinegar-
free, wheat-free, egg-free, dairy-free.

Barbara's Bakery
c/o Brewhurst [distributor]
A selection of dairy-free and wheat-
free cereal bars.

Barkat
c/o Gluten Free Foods Ltd [see below]
Gluten-free bread mixes; pizza crust
and breads free from gluten, wheat,
egg, milk and soya.

Bioferme
c/o NGT Associates [see below]
Selection of Yosa yoghurts made
from oats. Also available from
healthfood shops.

Blue Dragon Foods
c/o Suma Wholefoods [distributor]
Coconut milks, creamed coconut,
coconut powder, creamy coconut;
thick rice noodles; rice flour
pancakes; rice vinegar.

Bonsoy
c/o Brewhurst [distributor]
Soya milk.

Bute Island Foods
15 Columshill Street
Rothesay
Isle of Bute PA20 0HX
Tel: 01700 505 117
Dairy-free cheese alternatives.

Buxton Foods Ltd
12 Harley Street
London W1G 9PG
Tel: 020 7637 5505
Fax: 020 7436 0979
Website: www.stamp-
collection.co.uk
The Stamp Collection: dairy-free and
no-added-sugar chocolate with
sultana, apricot and sunflower
centres. Also hard and soft sheep's
cheeses, wheat-free pasta, bread,
flours and baking mixes. Vegetable
chips. Cookbook for special diets.
Available by mail order and in some
supermarkets and high street shops
nation-wide.

Clearspring Ltd
19A Acton Park Estate
London W3 7QE
Tel/Fax: 020 8749 1781
　　020 8746 0152 (for mail order)
Website: www.clearspring.co.uk
Dairy-free products; selection of rice cakes; gluten- and wheat-free foods; Japanese sauces, sea vegetables and teas. *Rice Dream*: a rice-based milk substitute; and *Imagine*: dairy-free desserts in various flavours. Available by mail order and from healthfood shops and supermarkets.

G Costa & Co. Ltd
Unit 6
Quarrywood Industrial Estate
Mills Road
Aylesford
Kent ME20 7NA
Tel: 01622 713 376
Fax: 01622 713 341
Website: www.gcosta.co.uk
Zest Foods vegan pesto and sun-dried tomato paste.

Daisy's Catering
Glandfield Cottage
Old School Mews
Sandgate
Kent CT20 3ST
Tel: 07050 136 179
Dairy-free fudge and assorted vegan fudge. Available by mail order (including in gift boxes).

Delamere Dairy
Yew Tree Farm
Bexton Lane
Knutsford
Cheshire WA16 9BA
Tel: 01565 632 422
Fax: 01565 750 468
Website: www.delamerediary.co.uk
Fresh and long-life goat's milk, yoghurt and cream, widely available through national retailers and by mail order.

Devon Fudge Direct
Unit 3
2A Barton Hill Road
Torquay
Devon TQ2 8JH
Tel/Fax: 01803 316 020
Website:
www.webstreet.co.uk/devonfudge
Excellent range of Radfords' assorted dairy-free coconut ice and fudge; walnut, ginger, chocolate, cherry, and rum & raisin.

Doves Farm Foods Ltd
Salisbury Road
Hungerford
Berkshire RG17 0RF
Tel: 01488 684 880
Website: www.dovesfarm.co.uk
Spelt, gram, maize, rice, buckwheat, rye and organic flours; vegan, dairy-free and soya-free digestive biscuits.

Dr Hadwen Trust
84A Tilehouse Street
Hitchin
Herts SG5 2DY
Tel: 01462 436 819
Fax: 01462 436 844
Website: www.drhadwentrust.org.uk
Large range of handmade adult and
children's chocolates, fudge, Turkish
delight, Christmas pudding, sweets,
truffles – all vegan, milk-free and egg-
free. Available only by mail order.

Ener-G Foods Inc.
c/o General Dietary Ltd [distributor]
Website: www.digimktg.com/energy
US company producing egg replacer
and a wide range of foods free from
wheat, gluten, dairy, soya, egg, corn,
etc. Rice bread and tapioca bread are
especially useful in exclusion diets
and for multiple allergies.

Everfresh Natural Foods
Gatehouse Close
Aylesbury
Bucks HP19 8DE
Tel: 01296 425 333
Fax: 01296 422 545
Website:
www.sunnyvale-organic.co.uk
Organic bread, cakes and puddings
free from yeast, milk, gluten, eggs
(and vegan): banana cake, chocolate
chip cake, fruit cake, stem ginger
cake, lemon cake, etc. Available at
healthfood shops and by mail order.

Evernat
c/o Brewhurst [distributor]
Organic milk drinks: almond,
hazelnut; and an organic range of
soya milk powder. All available from
healthfood shops.

Fabulous Foods
53 Lancaster Road
London N4 4PL
Tel: 020 7263 6989
Fax: 020 7263 5558
Selection of egg and egg-free noodles
from The Noodle Company. Mild
chilli and garlic ramen; medium
spinach noodles.

Fayrefield Foods Ltd
Englesea House
Barthomley Road
Crewe
Cheshire CW1 5UF
Tel: 01270 589 311
Fax: 01270 589 264
Website: www.fayrefield.com
Suppliers of non-dairy alternatives to
ice-cream (Swedish Glace) and full-
fat soft cheese (Swedish Soft). All
products are free from lactose and
cholesterol, and contain no
genetically modified ingredients.

First Foods
PO Box 140
Amersham
Bucks HP6 6XD
Tel: 01494 431 355
Fax: 01494 431 366
Website: www.first-foods.com
Products based on oats free from milk, dairy and soya. Oat milk, yoghurts and soft cheese and ice-creams in a variety of flavours. Available from major retailers and healthfood shops.

Galaxy Foods
c/o Brewhurst [distributors]
Dairy-free soya cheese slices. They also make rice cheese slices but these are *not* dairy-free as they contain casein.

General Dietary Ltd
PO Box 38
Kingston upon Thames
Surrey KT2 7YP
Tel: 020 8336 2323
Manufacturers of a variety of special diet products, including gluten-free breads and baguettes, rice breads, and pastas, egg replacer, biscuits, xantham gum, cereals, bread and pastry mixes that are free from wheat, soya, maize, gluten, egg, milk, lactose, casein and yeast. Available from any chemist dispensary and most healthfood shops. Associated brand names are *Ener-G, Valpiform* and *Tinkyada*.

Gluten Free Foods Ltd
Unit 270 Centennial Park
Centennial Avenue
Elstree
Borehamwood
Herts WD6 3SS
Tel: 020 8953 4444
Fax: 020 8953 8285
Website: www.glutenfree-foods.co.uk
Trades under the following names:
Glutano: gluten- and wheat-free biscuits, cakes, breads, bread mixes and pastas; selection of savoury snacks, pretzels and crackers. *Barkat*: rice breads, pizza crust, bread mix free from milk, yeast, gluten, wheat and egg.

Go Organic Ltd
24 Boswall Road
Edinburgh EH5 3RN
Tel/Fax: 0131 552 2706
Website: www.goorganic.co.uk
Curries, soups and sauces free from gluten, eggs and dairy products (some vegan). Available from healthfood shops and some supermarkets.

Granovita UK Ltd
5 Stanton Close
Finedon Road Industrial Estate
Wellingborough
Northants NN8 4HN
Tel: 01933 273 717
Fax: 01933 273 3729
Website: www.granovita.co.uk
Full range of products suitable for dairy-free and gluten-free diets; soya milks; *Soyage* yoghurts in various flavours. Yeast and vegetable spreads. Various organic vegetable patés, and fruit and vegetable juices. Egg-free mayonnaise. Fruit bars. Many products are vegan, so suitable for diets free from dairy, egg and fish. Available at healthfood shops and some supermarkets.

Haldane Foods Group
Howard Way
Newport Pagnall
Bucks MK16 9PY
Tel: 01908 211 311
Fax: 01908 210 514
Website: www.haldane.co.uk
Vegetarian and vegan foods under brand names *Granose*, *Realeat*, *Organic* and *Direct Foods*. Includes a range of organic dairy-free ice delight, soya milks, cream, yoghurts, snack pots and frozen meals in a variety of flavours. Widely available.

Itona Products
Wigan
WN1 2SB
Granny Ann beanmilk chunky 'chocolate' eggs and gluten-free biscuits. Send s.a.e. for information.

Juvela
SHS International Ltd
100 Wavertree Boulevard
Wavertree Technology Park
Liverpool L7 9PT
Tel: 0151 228 8161
Fax: 0151 228 2650
Website: www.shsweb.co.uk
A selection of gluten-free breads, bread mixes, biscuits and crackers, available at pharmacies/chemists and on prescription.

Kallo Foods
Coopers Place
Coombe Lane
Wormley
Surrey GU8 5SZ
Tel: 01428 685 100
Fax: 01428 685 800
Fromsoya: non-dairy cheese spreads in a variety of flavours. A selection of rice cakes.

Kinnerton (Confectionery) Co. Ltd
49 Marylebone High Street
London W1W 5EB
Tel: 020 7470 1914
Fax: 020 7470 1810
Website: www.kinnerton.com
Have separated their factory into nut and nut-free zones, so their nut-free chocolate is guaranteed to be nut-free. Catalogue available for children's novelty bars, Easter eggs and a Christmas selection. Widely available.

Lifestyle Healthcare Ltd
Centenary Business Park
Henley-on-Thames RG9 1DS
Tel: 01491 411 767
Fax: 01491 570 001
Website: www.gfdiet.com
A selection of biscuits free from
gluten, wheat and milk. Gluten-free
breads, fruit buns, rolls, puddings,
sweet and savoury pastry goods, all
freshly cooked. Available on
prescription at pharmacies/chemists.
Home deliveries throughout the UK.

Linda McCartney Vegetarian Foods
(owned by H J Heinz)
Tel: 0800 626 697
'Yoghurt' and soya-based frozen
desserts.

Lyme Regis Fine Foods Ltd
Station Industrial Estate
Liphook
Hampshire GU30 7DR
Tel: 01428 722 900
Fax: 01428 727 222
Website: www.lyme-regis-foods.com
Range of snacks free from wheat,
milk and sugar; fruit bars; chocolate-
coated marzipan bar. From
healthfood shops, direct by mail
order or from a wholesaler.

Matthews Foods plc
The Healy Complex
Healy Road
Ossett
West Yorkshire WF5 8NE
Tel: 01924 272 534
Fax: 01924 277 071
Website: www.purespreads.com
Manufacturers of *Pure* dairy-free
sunflower spread, soya spread and
organic spread.

Meridian Foods Ltd
Corwen
Derbyshire LL21 9RJ
Manufacturers of soya margarine.

Morehands Ltd
c/o AllergyFree Direct [distributors]
Florentino Parmazano non-animal
dairy/milk/egg-free Parmesan-style
'cheese'.

Mrs Leeper's Gourmet Pasta
c/o Brewhurst [distributors]
Corn and rice pastas free from wheat
and gluten.

New Nutrition
Woodlands
London Road
Battle
E Sussex TN33 0LP
Tel: 01424 774 103
Fax: 01424 775 200
Whole-egg replacer and Arise, a
raising agent for yeast-free breads,
are just two of a whole range of
special dietary products. Available
only by mail order.

NGT Associates
Unit 23
Bardfield Centre
Braintree Road
Great Bardfield
Essex CM7 4SL
Tel: 01371 811 134
Fax: 01371 811 194
Website: www.ngtassociates.co.uk
UK agent for *Yosa* dairy- and soya-free yoghurt-type snack with 'friendly' bacteria: fruits of the forest, peach & passion fruit, pineapple, apple & banana – with added calcium. Also a distributor for *Lyme Regis Foods* and *Panda Foods*. Available at healthfood shops and some supermarkets.

Norfolk Truffle Company
Hall Farm
Bungay Road
Morningthorpe
Norfolk NR15 2LJ
Dairy-free organic range of truffles. Note that some contain nuts.

Nutricia Dietary Care
Newmarket Avenue
White Horse Business Park
Trowbridge
Wiltshire BA14 0XQ
Tel: 01225 711 801
Fax: 01225 711 567
Website: www.glutafin.co.uk
A variety of products free from gluten, wheat, milk and egg. *Rite Diet*: breads, rolls, baking powder and flour mixes. *Glutafin*: large variety of bread, cakes, mixes, biscuits, pizza bases and baguettes. Available on prescription at pharmacies/chemist shops.

Nutrition Point Ltd
13 Taurus Park
Westbrook
Warrington WA5 5ZT
Tel: 07041 544 044
Fax: 07041 544 055
Website:
www.dietaryspecialties.co.uk
A large selection of bread, cake, scone and pastry mixes free from wheat and gluten. Recipe cards available on request.

Organic Supplies Company
Valleycraft Ltd
65 Saddleback Road
Camberley
Surrey GU15 4DA
Tel/Fax: 01276 684 604
Import *Sojami* products which are soya-based, dairy-free and vegan. Spreads: garlic-thyme, garlic-basil, chives-shallot, cumin-tarragon, garlic & herb, garlic-pepper, seaweeds, green olive, black olive, curry, sesame, and a vegan crème fraiche.

Orgran
c/o Community Foods [distributor]
Website: www.orgran.com
Whole-egg-replacer and a wide range of wheat- and gluten-free products, including pastas, fruit bars, pancake mix, gravy mix, pizza mix, falafel mix, corn cakes, rice cakes, crispbreads and spaghetti in tomato sauce.

Pamela's
c/o Brewhurst [distributor]
Tel: 01932 334 501
A variety of gluten-free biscuits:
pecan shortbread, butter shortbread,
ginger cookies, shortbread swirl,
peanut butter cookies, lemon
shortbread, carob hazelnut cookies,
simply chocolate shortbread.
Available at healthfood shops.

Peter Moxham Trading
Cornwallis House
Howard Chase
Basildon
Essex SS14 3BB
Tel: 01268 286 341
Fax: 01268 281 193
Fruit bars free from milk, egg, wheat,
gluten, soya, maize and most other
things! Flavours: apple & apricot,
raspberry, strawberry, wildberry,
cherry, blueberry, apple, tutti frutti.
Available at independent healthfood
shops.

Plamil Foods
Plamil House
4 Bowles Well Gardens
Dover Road
Folkestone
Kent CT19 6PQ
Tel: 01303 850 588
Fax: 01303 850 015
Website: www.plamilfoods.co.uk
Variety of dairy-free chocolates:
plain, milk and flavoured. Carob
drops. Dairy-free milk, cream, etc.
Egg-free mayonnaise: plain, garlic,
tarragon, organic. Organic sandwich
spreads: paprika (soya-free),
vegetable (gluten- and yeast-free),
tofu plus curry and pineapple (soya-
free). Soya products. Also runs the
British Alternative Milk Advisory
Service.

Plas Farm Ltd
Celtic House
Gaerwen
Anglesey LL60 6HR
Tel: 01248 422 011
Fax: 01248 422 003
Manufacturers of egg-free
mayonnaise, coleslaw and *Biddy
Merkins* brand Vegerella dairy-free
cheese substitute (also gluten- and
soya-free and vegan). Available from
healthfood shops.

Pleniday
c/o Brewhurst [distributor]
Tel: 01932 334 501
Large range of gluten-free products,
including low-fat varieties. Biscuits
include: chocolate chip crunch,
coconut crunch, ginger nut and
sultana spice. Cakes, crispy bars,
muesli-flavoured mini rice cakes,
bread mixes, cake mixes, pastas.
Many lines on prescription.

Prosoya
2–5310 Canotek Road
Ottowa
Ontario K1J 9N5
Canada
Tel: (Canada) 613 745 9115
Fax: (Canada) 613 745 2045
Website: www.prosoya.ca
SoNice brand of soya milks

Provamel
see Vandermoortele (UK) Ltd

Pure Wine Co.
Unit 18
Woods Browning Industrial Estate
Respryn Road
Bodmin PL31 1DQ
Tel: 01208 79300
Fax: 01208 79393
Website: www.purewine.co.uk
Selection of organic wines that are
vegan (i.e. not clarified with any egg,
milk or fish products). Available by
mail order and to trade.

R J Foods Ltd
Units 1–4
7 Airfield Road
Airfield Industrial estate
Christchurch
Dorset BH23 3TQ
Tel/Fax: 01202 481 471
Vegan (free from milk, eggs, animal
products) fruit bars and flapjacks;
vegetarian fruit bars, flapjacks and
individually wrapped cookies (some
vegan).

Rakusen's
Rakusen House
Clayton Wood Rise
Ring Road, West Park
Leeds
W Yorks LS16 6QN
Tel: 0113 278 4821
Fax: 0113 278 4064
Website: www.rakusens.co.uk
Dairy-free margarine Tomor. Also a
selection of kosher foods that are
dairy-free, including non-dairy ice-
creams. Vegetable and/or soya based.
Widely available.

Redwood Wholefood Company
Redwood House
60 Burkitt Road
Corby
Northants NN17 4DT
Tel: 01536 400 557
Fax: 01536 408 878
Website: www.redwoodfoods.co.uk
Large selection of vegan foods,
including the Cheezly selection of
alternative cheeses. All suitable for
egg-free and milk-free diets.

Rich Products Ltd
Rough Farm
Atherstone on Stour
Stratford upon Avon
Warwickshire CV37 8DX
Tel: 01789 450 030
Whip topping 'cream'

Scanian Farmers
21 Sercombe Park
Clevedon
N Somerset BS21 5BA
Tel: 01275 794 063
Website: www.oatly.com
Organic dairy and genetically
modified-free oat-based milk (Oatly)
from Sweden. Available from
Waitrose and other supermarkets.

Schär
PO Box 126
Worcester WR5 2ZN
Tel/Fax: 01905 357 899
Customer line: 0808 1000 483
A good selection of products free
from wheat and gluten, many of
which are available on prescription.
Includes Schär biscuits, pastas,
bread, rolls, crispbreads, crackers
and cakes.

Scientific Hospital Supplies (SHS)
100 Wavertree Boulevard
Wavertree Technology Park
Liverpool L7 9PT
Tel: 0151 228 1992
Fax: 0151 228 2650
Website: www.shsweb.co.uk
Manufacture the *Juvela* range of
wheat-free and gluten-free products,
many of which are available on
prescription.

Shepherd Boy
Healthcross House
Cross Street
Syston
Leicester LE7 2JG
Tel: 0116 260 2992
Fax: 0116 269 3106
Website: www.shepherdboy.uk
Just So carob bars: crispy, orange,
peppermint, ginger – free from milk,
egg and animal products (vegan).
Also fruit, nut and seed bars; muesli;
hemp oil capsules (similar to cod liver
oil; contain omega 3 and 6).

Skane Dairy UK
21 Sercombe Park
Clevedon
N Somerset BS21 5BA
Tel: 01275 794 063
Helpline: 0845 6011 754
Fax: 01275 794 066
Website: www.proviva.com
Non-dairy probiotic fruit drink
(*Proviva*).

Smilde Food Group
PO Box 27
Crowborough
E Sussex TN6 3SF
Tel: 01892 669 616
Fax:01892 669 617
Website: www.smildefood.uk.com
Bebo vegan sunflower spreads.

SoGood International
Stuart House
City Road
Peterborough PE1 1QF
Customer Careline 0800 328 0423
Fax: 01892 512 903
Website: www.sogood123.com
SoGood range of soya beverages,
available from most supermarkets
and healthfood stores.

Sojasun
c/o Windmill Organics [distributor]
Selection of soya-based dairy-free
vegan yoghurts, desserts, milks,
available from healthfood shops and
most wholesalers.

Soya Health Foods Ltd
Station House
Stamford New Road
Altrincham
Cheshire WA14 1EP
Tel: 0161 924 2214
Fax: 0161 924 2213
Sunrise: no-added-sugar soya milk
drinks and powders; dairy-free choc
ices.

Stiletto Foods
Tennyson House
Tennyson Road
London W7 1LH
Tel: 020 8840 2244
Mrs Crimble's cakes free from egg and
wheat.

Sun Foods
Van Guard Trading Centre
16 Marshgate Lane
London E15 2NH
Tel: 020 8555 7075
A variety of cakes and breads free
from eggs, gluten, wheat and dairy.

Sussex High Weald Dairy
Putlands Farm
Duddleswell
Uckfield
E Sussex TN22 3BJ
Tel: 01825 712 647
Fax: 01825 712 477
Website: www.specialty-foods.com
Dairy sheep products: milk, fromage
frais, yoghurt, a hard cheese, soft
cheeses, feta, halloumi and ricotta;
cheeses from organic cows. Available
by mail order and stocked nationally
at delicatessens, farm shops and farm
markets.

Tofutti UK Ltd
5th floor, Congress House
14 Lyon Road
Harrow
Middx HA1 2FD
Tel: 020 8861 4443
Fax: 020 8861 0444
Website: www.trianobrands.co.uk
Snowcrest 'cream' whip; luxurious
dairy-free ice-cream and cheese
spreads.

Traidcraft plc
Kingsway
Gateshead
Tyne & Wear NE11 0NE
Tel: 0191 491 0591
Fax: 0191 482 2690
Website: www.traidcraft.co.uk
Continental dairy-free chocolate.
Available by mail order or through
healthfood stores.

Trufree
Newmarket Avenue
White Horse Business Park
Trowbridge
Wiltshire BA14 0XQ
Tel: 01225 711 801
Orderline: 0870 241 3919
Fax: 01225 711 567
Website: www.trufree.co.uk
Range of products free from gluten,
wheat, milk and egg: white rolls,
white loaf, part-baked rolls and
bread, cake and pastry mixes.
Biscuits and quick snacks (similar to
Pot Noodle). Available at healthfood
shops and by mail order.

Ultrapharm
Centennial Business Park
Henley-on-Thames
Oxon RG9 1DS
Tel: 01491 570 000
Fax: 01491 570 001
Website: www.gfdiet.com
Gluten-free bakers with a wide range
of breads, cakes, crackers and
biscuits, available on prescription
and by mail order as *Lifestyle
Products*. Also own *Allergycare* –
dairy-free confectionery; alternative
milks; cooking aids; gluten-free gravy
powder, baking powder and stuffing
mix. Whole-egg replacer.

Vandermoortele (UK) Ltd
Ashley House
86–94 High Street
Hounslow
Middx TW3 1NH
Tel: 020 8814 7826
Fax: 020 8577 7441
Websites: www.provamel.co.uk
www.sojanet.com
Wide range of non-dairy creams,
yoghurts, desserts and ice-creams,
available in most supermarkets and
healthfood shops. Range of soya
milks: calcium-enriched, sweetened
and unsweetened, with added
vitamins and minerals, organic;
lunch box size: banana, strawberry,
chocolate; 330 ml soya fruity
(milk/juice mix) in various flavours.

Vegan Cake Company
Tel: 020 7243 8225
Mobile: 0771 200 6983
Individually designed vegan cakes
(egg-, dairy-, animal-free) made to
order. (Address – in Notting Hill,
London – given only for customers to
collect their orders.)

Vermont Nutfree Chocolates
316 Route 2
PO Box 124
South Hero
VT 05486
U S A
Tel: [US] 802 372 4654
1-888-4-NUT-FREE
Website: www.vermontnutfree.com
Supplier of peanut/nut-free
chocolates, including truffles, fruit
creams, mint creams, caramels,
clusters, assortments, milk/dark
bars, minibars, chocolate drops,
novelty lollipops, bugs and chocolate
coins.

Village Bakery
Melmerby
Penrith
Cumbria CA10 1HE
Tel: 01768 881 515
Fax: 01768 881 848
Website: www.village-bakery.com
Special diet products on mail order,
including products free from wheat,
yeast, dairy, sugar and salt. Bread,
biscuits and cakes. New selection of
Christmas products suitable for
wheat- and gluten-free diets. Also a
good selection of vegan cakes,
biscuits and slices. Available by mail
order or through selected stockists
(list of stockists available).

Vinceremos Wines & Spirits
19 New Street
Leeds LS18 4BH
Tel: 0113 205 4545
Fax: 0113 205 4546
Website: www.vinceremos.co.uk
Suppliers of vegan (milk- and egg-
free) and organic wines and low-
sulphur wines.

Vintage Roots Ltd
Farley Farms/Bridge Farm
Reading Road
Arborfield
Berks RG2 9HT
Tel: 0118 976 1999
Freephone 0800 980 4992
Fax: 0118 976 1998
Website: www.vintageroots.co.uk
Vegan, organic and low-sulphur
wines, spirits and beers, available by
mail order or at selected healthfood
shops and specialist off-licences.

Vitaquell
c/o Brewhurst [distributor]
Various dairy-free margarines.

Vitariz
c/o Health Store or Suma
[distributors]
Organic rice drink made in Italy and
distributed via the wholesalers.
Available direct from the wholesaler
or from healthfood shops.

Vitasoy
c/o Brewhursts [distributor]
Soya milk.

Viva!
12 Queen Square
Brighton BN1 3FD
Tel: 01273 777 688
Fax: 01273 776 755
Website: www.viva.org.uk
Vegan organisation selling dairy-free fudge, chocolate beans and chocolate in bars and boxes. Available only by mail order. Also a good selection of vegan cookery books.

Whole Earth Foods Ltd
2 Valentine Place
London SE1 8QH
Tel: 020 7633 5900
Fax: 020 7633 5901/2
Websites:
www.wholeearthfoods.com
www.greenandblacks.com
Variety of organic dairy-free, gluten-free cereals and chocolate (chocolate under the name *Green & Black's*). You should read the individual products labels to check for their suitability for your diet; not all their chocolate is dairy-free. Free recipe booklet on request. Widely available, and via mail order.

INFANT NUTRITION

Cow & Gate Nutricia Ltd
White Horse Business Park
Trowbridge
Wiltshire BA14 0XQ
Tel: 01225 768 381
Babyfeeding information service:
08457 623 623
Fax: 01225 768 847
Milupa and *Cow & Gate* formulas and baby foods.

Farley's and Heinz
H J Heinz Co Ltd
6 South Building
Hayes Park
Hayes
Middx UB4 8AL
Tel: 020 8573 7757
Farley's Careline: 0845 057 0057
(info on formulas Mon–Fri 8.30 a.m.–5.30 p.m.)
Fax: 020 8848 2325
Website: www.heinz.co.uk
Make a variety of (Farley's) formula milks and (Heinz) baby foods.

Mead Johnson Nutritionals
141–149 Staines Road
Hounslow
Middx TW3 3JA
Tel: 020 8754 3764
Fax: 020 8569 5091
Make a variety of formula milks and baby foods, available on prescription and over the counter.

SHS International Ltd
100 Wavertree Boulevard
Wavertree Technology Park
Liverpool L7 9PT
Tel: 0151 228 8161
Fax: 0151 228 2650
Website: www.shsweb.co.uk
Make *Neocate* elemental infant
formula (available only on
prescription) as well as *Juvela* gluten-
free and dairy-free products.

SMA Nutrition
Huntercombe Lane South
Taplow
Maidenhead
Berks SL6 0PH
Tel: 0345 762 900
Fax: 01628 604 949
Website: www.wyeth.co.uk
Make a variety of formula and
specialist milks. Available on
prescription and over the counter.

Vitacare Ltd
Unit 1
7 Chalcot Road
Primrose Hill
London NW1 8LH
Tel: 020 7722 4300
Helpline: 0800 328 5826
Fax: 020 7722 7737
Website: www.vitacare.co.uk
Nanny: goat's milk complete infant
nutrition formula. Free from soya,
nuts and cow's milk. Used for
eczema, asthma, infant colic and
cow's milk intolerance. Call Helpline
for stockists and more information.

OTHER FOOD MANUFACTURERS

Bart Spices Ltd
Bristol BS3 4AD
Coconut milk, and organically grown
herbs and spices.

Birds Eye Frozen Foods
Station Avenue
Walton-on-Thames
Surrey KT12 1NT
Tel: 01932 263 177
Freephone 0800 33 22 77
Websites:
www.captainbirdseye.co.uk (for
children)
www.unilever.com
'Free from' lists for various special
diets available on request.

Cadbury Trebor Bassett Ltd
Consumer Services
PO Box 7009
Bourneville
Birmingham B30 2LU
Tel: 0121 451 4444
'Free from' lists for various special
diets available on request.

Golden Wonder Ltd
Edinburgh House
Abbey Street
Market Harborough
Leics LE16 9AA
Tel: 01858 461 000
Fax: 01858 414 110
'Free from' lists for various special
diets available on request.

H J Heinz
Department of Nutrition
Kitt Green
Wigan
Lancs WN5 0JL
Tel: 01942 624 374
Website: www.heinz.co.uk
'Free from' lists for various special
diets available on request.

Kellogg's Co. GB Ltd
Consumer Services
Kellogg Building
Talbot Road
Manchester M16 0PU
Tel: 0161 869 2000
        0800 626 066 (advice)
Fax: 0161 869 2103
Website: www.kelloggs.co.uk
'Free from' lists for various special
diets available on request.

Lindt & Sprüngli (UK) Ltd
Stockley road
West Drayton
Middx UB7 9BG
Importers of the Lindt brand of Swiss
chocolates

Mars Confectionery
Dundee Road
Slough SL1 4JX
Tel: 01753 550 055
Fax: 01753 550 111
Website: www.snickers.com
'Free from' lists for various special
diets available on request.

McVities (UK)
Watermans Business Park
The Causeway
Staines
Middx TW18 3BA
Tel: 01784 447744
Careline: 0500 011 710
Fax: 01784 447 711
Website: www.unitedbiscuits.com
'Free from' lists for various special
diets available on request.

Nestlé UK Ltd
Consumer Services
PO Box 203
York YO91 1XY
Tel: 0800 000 030
Fax: 01904 603 461
Website: www.nestle.co.uk
Produce literature on nut-free diets
and a 'free from nuts' list. Labelling
initiatives to include nuts if they are
an ingredient, in any form. Makers of
After Eight chocolates.

Thorntons plc
Thornton Park
Somercotes
Alfreton
Derbyshire DE55 4XJ
Tel: 01773 540 550
Helpline: 01773 542 059
Fax: 01773 540 757
Website: www.thorntons.co.uk
'Free from' lists for various special
diets available on request. Also
seasonal lists for Easter, Mother's
Day, Christmas, etc., on request.

Van den Bergh Foods Ltd
Crawley RH10 2RQ
Makers of *Flora* margarines.

Walkers Snack Foods Ltd
Feature Road
Thurmaston
Leicester LE4 8BS
Tel: 0116 234 2345
Fax: 0116 234 2340
Website: www.walkers.co.uk
'Free from' lists available, on request,
for all the major allergens.

Walls
Station Avenue
Walton-on-Thames
Surrey KT12 1NT
Tel: 0800 731 1507
Website: www.unilever.com
'Free from' lists for various special
diets available on request.

Weetabix Ltd
Station Road
Burton Latimer
Northants NN15 5JR
Tel: 01536 722 181
Fax: 01536 726 148
'Free from' lists for various special
diets available on request.

DISTRIBUTORS OF SPECIAL DIET PRODUCTS
(also called wholesalers or suppliers)

AllergyFree Direct Ltd
5 Centremead
Osney Mead
Oxford OX2 0ES
Tel: 01865 722 003
Fax: 01865 244 134
Website: www.allergyfreedirect.co.uk
Mail order specialist for foods free
from wheat, gluten, milk and egg;
vegan and vegetarian foods also
available. The website is easy to
navigate with the categories clearly
labelled and giving the ingredients
used for each product. It also
contains a glossary.

Brewhurst Health Food Supplies Ltd
Abbot Close
Oyster Lane
Byfleet
Surrey KT14 7JP
Tel: 01932 354 211
Fax: 01932 336 235
Website: www.brewhurst.com
Distributor of a wide range of
products for special diets, including
Galaxy Foods (soya cheese slices), *Mrs
Leeper's* (wheat- and gluten-free
pasta), *Pamela's* (wheat- and gluten-
free biscuits), *Pleniday* (gluten-free
products), *Vitaquell* and *Vitasoy*. And
many others.

Community Foods Ltd
Micross
Brent Terrace
London NW2 1LT
Tel: 020 8450 9411
Fax: 020 8208 1803
Website:
www.communityfoods.co.uk
Pasta, pancake mixes, tinned
spaghetti, fruit bars free from wheat
and gluten. Dairy-free chocolates.
Agent for *Orgran* (egg-replacer) and
Tropical Source dairy-free chocolate
bars in six flavours.

De Rit (UK) Ltd
Tenterfields Business Park
Luddendenfoot
Halifax HX2 6EJ
Tel: 01422 885 523
Fax: 01422 884 629
Own range of products imported
from Holland and distributor for
other products, including *Orgran*
wheat- and gluten-free pastas.

Fairhaven Wholefoods Ltd
27 Jubilee Trade Centre
Letchworth
Herts SG6 1SP
Tel: 01462 675 300
Fax: 01462 483 008
Website: www.fairhaven.co.uk
Shop and wholefood supplier selling
a good selection of foods suitable for
special diets.

Good Food Distributors
Unit 35
Ddole Road Industrial Estate
Llandrindod Wells
Powys LD1 6DF
Tel: 01597 824 720
       0800 833 068 (orderline)
Fax: 01597 824 760
Website:
www.goodfooddistributors.co.uk
Distributor of a good selection of
food suitable for special diets.

Goodness Direct
South March
Daventry
Northants NN11 4PH
Tel: 01327 871 655
Fax: 01327 300 436
Website: www.GoodnessDirect.co.uk
Distributor of a range of products
suitable for special diets.

Health Store
Bastow House
Queens Road
Nottingham NG2 3AS
Tel: 0115 955 5255
Careline: 0800 952 0023
Fax: 0115 955 5290
Distributor for a very wide range of
healthfoods, supplements and
products suitable for all types of
special diets.

Infinity Foods Co-operative Ltd
67 Norway Street
Portslade
E Sussex BN41 1AE
Tel: 01273 424 060
Fax: 01273 417 739
Organic food wholesaler and
distributor selling products suitable
for all special diets.

Marigold Healthfoods Ltd
102 Camley Street
London NW1 0PF
Tel: 020 7388 4515
Fax: 020 7388 4516
Distributor for *Engevita* nutritional
yeast flakes that can be used as a
cheese substitute to sprinkle on pizza,
pasta, etc., and a variety of bouillon
powders that are suitable for diets
free from yeast, wheat, gluten, soya,
egg and cow's milk. Many other lines
also available.

Suma Wholefoods
Unit AX1
Dean Clough Industrial Park
Halifax
W Yorkshire HX3 5AN
Tel: 01422 345 513
Fax: 01422 349 429
Website: www.suma.co.uk
A distributor of other companies'
products but also has its own brands.
All are vegetarian; some are vegan
and organic. A range of dairy-free
and soya-free full-fat and low-fat
spreads. *Vegannaise*: egg-free
mayonnaise. Some soups are free
from gluten, milk, egg and soya;
dairy-free pesto; and much, much
more.

Windmill Organics
Unit 4, Atlas Transport Estate
Bridges Court, off York Road
London SW11 3QS
Tel: 020 7924 2300
Fax: 020 7223 8370
Wholesaler for organic foods,
including many that are suitable for
special diets. *Biona Foods* for wheat-
and gluten-free cookies, cakes,
pastas, breads, mixes. Vegan spreads
free from dairy and soya. *Rapunzel*
Swiss chocolate.

FOOD OUTLETS

Beefeater
Whitbread plc
Whitbread House
Park Street West
Luton
Beds LU1 3BG
Tel: 01582 844300
Website: www.beefeater.co.uk
For a list of ingredients contained in
food served at its restaurants.

Burger King Ltd
Charter Place
Vine Street
Uxbridge
Middx UB8 1BZ
Tel: 01895 206000
Fax: 01895 206026
Website: www.burgerking.com
For a list of ingredients contained in
food served at its restaurants.

McDonald's Restaurants Ltd
11–59 High Road
East Finchley
London N2 8AW
Tel: 0990 244622 (customer care)
Fax: 020 8700 7060
Website: www.mcdonalds.com
For a list of ingredients contained in
food served at its restaurants.

Pizza Hut UK Ltd
1 Imperial Place
Elstree Way
Borehamwood
Herts WD6 1JN
Tel: 020 8732 9000
Fax: 020 8732 9009
Website: www.pizzahut.co.uk
For a list of ingredients contained in
food served at its restaurants.

Pret à Manger
16 Palace Street
London SW1E 5PT
Tel: 020 7827 8000
Fax: 020 7827 8787
Website: www.pret.com
For a list of ingredients contained in
food served at its restaurants.

SUPERMARKETS AND STORES

Asda
Customer Services Department
Asda House
Great Wilson Street
Leeds LS11 5AD
Tel: 0113 243 5435
Freephone: 0500 10 00 55
Website: www.asda.co.uk
'Free from' booklets available on request.

Boots Customer Services
PO Box 5300
Nottingham NG90 1AA
Tel: 0845 070 8090
Fax: 0115 959 5525
Website: www.boots.co.uk
Will provide, on request, 'free from' lists on their own-brand products. Also produce infant formulas.

Co-op
Customer Services
CWS Ltd
Freepost MR9 473
Manchester M4 8BA
Tel: 0800 0686 727; 0800 317 827
Fax: 0161 827 6604
Website: www. co-op.co.uk
Will provide, on request, 'free from' lists free of charge for their own-brand products.

Marks and Spencer
Customer Services, Room 101
27 Baker Street
London W1V 8EP
Tel: 020 7268 1234
Fax: 020 7268 2380
Website: www.marksandspencer.com
Will provide, on request, information on own-brand foods that are suitable for special diets.

Safeway plc
Customer Services
Beddow Way
Aylesford
Maidstone
Kent ME20 7AT
Tel: 01622 712 546
Fax: 01622 712 160/712 111
Website: www.safeway.co.uk
Will provide, on request, information on own-brand products that are suitable for special diets. (This information is also available on the actual product labels.)

J Sainsbury plc
Customer Services
Stamford House
London SE1 9LL
Tel: 0800 636 262
Fax: 020 7695 7765
Website: www.sainsbury.co.uk
'Free from' lists for various special diets available on request.

Somerfield Stores Ltd
Customer Relations/Services
Somerfield House
Whitchurch Lane
Bristol BS14 0TJ
Tel: 0117 935 9359
Fax: 0117 978 0629
Website: www.somerfield.co.uk
'Free from' lists for various special
diets available on request.

Tesco
Customer Service Centre
Box 73
Baird Avenue
Dundee DD1 9NF
Helpline: 0800 505 555
Fax: 01382 819 956
Website: www.tesco.co.uk
'Free from' lists for various special
diets available on request.

Waitrose
Nutritional Advice Centre
Waitrose
Southern Industrial Area
Bracknell
Berks RG12 8YA
Tel: 01344 824 975
Fax: 01344 825 297/824 990
Website: www.waitrose.co.uk
'Free from' lists for various special
diets available on request.

SPECIAL DIET COOKERY COURSES

As well as the courses listed below,
enquire at your local college – they
may run a course or know of one
elsewhere.

Catering Imaginaire
12 Priory Walk
St Albans
Herts AL1 2JA
Roselyne Masselin (director),
a creative cookery writer and
demonstrator, teaches vegan cookery
and the use of vegan products and
recipes.

Leaves of Life
51 Gladesmore Road
London N15 6TA
Tel/Fax: 020 8800 1850
Website: leavesoflife.org
Vegetarian/vegan cookery
demonstrations.

Penrhos Court
Kington
Herefordshire HR5 3LH
Tel: 01544 230 720
Fax: 01544 230 754
Websites: www.penrhos.co.uk
www.greencuisine.org
Special diet cookery courses available
at school in beautiful surroundings,
using only organic food.

Ploughshares Training
54 Roman Way
Glastonbury
Somerset BA6 8AD
Tel/Fax: 01458 831 182
Staff will teach you how to cook for a special diet in the comfort of your own home.

ACCOMMODATION AND EATING OUT

Note that all the vegan premises welcome vegans and non-vegans alike.

Bay Tree
403 Great Western Road
Glasgow G4 9HY
Tel: 01413 345 898
Vegan café with a Middle Eastern style.

Beachcroft Hotel & Restaurant
Clyde Road
Felpham
Bognor Regis PO22 7AH
Tel: 01243 827 142
Happy to accommodate special dietary requirements if contact is made in advance to explain special needs.

Birchtrees
Reiffer Park Road
Sorbie
Wigtownshire DG8 8EH
Tel: 01988 850 391
B&B catering for special diets on request.

Brambles
10 Clarence Road
Shanklin
PO37 7BH
Tel: 01983 862 507
Vegan guest house, therefore guaranteed free from eggs, milk and dairy, fish, shellfish and meat. Run by John and Mary Anderson. (5 minutes to the nearest sandy beach!)

Chi (was **Veg Chinese Veg Restaurant**)
8 Egerton Gardens Mews
Knightsbridge
London SW3 2EH
Tel: 020 7584 7007
Fantastic vegan Chinese. All food is
100% free of meat, fish, shellfish,
egg, milk and dairy products.

Fisher King Centre
54 Roman Way
Glastonbury BA6 8AD
Tel/Fax: 01458 831182
B&B of vegan organic cuisine. Also
available: shiatsu, special diet/vegan
courses, deep cleansing programme.

Fox Hall
Sedgwick
Kendal
Cumbria LA8 0JP
Tel/Fax: 015395 61241
Website:
www.fox.hall.btinternet.co.uk
Vegan B&B. Food guaranteed to be
free from meat, fish, shellfish, eggs,
milk and dairy products (proprietors
are called Sylvia and Chris).

Greenacres Country Guesthouse
Lindale
Grange-over-Sands
Cumbria LA11 6LP
Tel/Fax: 015395 34578
Licensed guesthouse. The proprietor,
Barbara, has cooked gluten-free
meals for the past 20 years for a
family member. She used to work as a
special diet chef in a hospital kitchen
so she has an excellent knowledge of
special diets. She is happy to provide
special dietary meals on request.
Menus also printed in Braille.

Greenbanks Hotel
Swaffham Road
Wendling
Norwich NR19 2AB
Tel: 01362 687742
Website:
www.greenbankshotel.co.uk
Proprietor, Jennie Lock, provides
home-produced gluten-free and
vegan food and caters for other
special diets on request. Braille
menus.

Heathers
74 McMillan Street
London SE8 3HA
Tel: 020 8691 6665
Fax: 020 8692 3263
Website: www.heathers.dircon.co.uk
Vegan and vegetarian restaurant,
also offering food free from milk and
egg. Happy to cater for other special
diets on request.

Making Waves
3 Richmond Place
St Ives
Cornwall TR26 1JN
Tel: 01736 793 895
Website: www.making-waves.co.uk
Rustic vegan guesthouse. Food is
guaranteed 100% free from meat,
fish, shellfish, eggs, milk and dairy
products. Can also provide nut-,
wheat- and gluten-free food on
request. Friendly and helpful
proprietor called Simon.

Middle Rylands
Redmoor
Bodmin
Cornwall PL30 5AR
Tel: 01208 872 316
Vegan B&B in beautiful
surroundings, run by Joan Dell.

Penrhos Court
Kington
Herefordshire HR5 3LH
Tel: 01544 230 720
Fax: 01544 230 754
Websites: www.penrhos.co.uk
www.greencuisine.org
Hotel that caters for people with
special diets.

Queenswood Hotel
Victoria Park
Weston-super-Mare BS23 2HZ
Tel: 01934 416 141
Fax: 01934 621 759
Website: www.queenswoodhotel.com
Run by Margaret and David Horler,
who have first-hand experience of
various food allergies. Many special
diets catered for by arrangement.

Rossan Guest House
Auchencairn
Castle Douglas
Kirkcudbrightshire DG7 1QR
Tel: 01556 640 269
Fax: 01556 640 278
e-mail: bardsley@rossan.freeserve.co
Website: www.SmoothHound.co.uk/
hotels/rossan.html
Bed, breakfast and evening meal
available. Delightful proprietor, Mrs
Bardsley, offers food for all special
diets on request. Picnics provided.
Dogs free.

Stonecroft
Edale
Hope Valley
Derbyshire S33 7ZA
Website:www.cressbrook.co.uk/
edale/stonecroft
Tel/Fax: 01433 670 262
Guest house catering for all special
diets. The proprietor, Julia, has an
excellent understanding of
anaphylaxis and cross-
contamination issues. She is coeliac
herself and follows a strict gluten-
and wheat-free diet. Bed, breakfast
and evening meals, long and short
stays available.

13th Note
50–60 King Street
Glasgow G1 5QT
Tel: 0141 553 1638
Fax: 0141 400 1638
Website: www.13thnote.com.uk
All-vegan café/bar with occasional
gigs. Wide range of food, including
their famous dairy-free cheesecake.
Dance it off afterwards at the 13th
Note Club in Clyde Street.

Trewella Guest House
18 Mennaye Road
Penzance
Cornwall TR18 4NG
Tel: 01736 363818
Special diets catered for. Only bed and
breakfast available. Proprietors are
Shan and Dave Glenn.

Westwood Country Hotel
Hinksey Hilltop
Oxford OX1 5BG
Tel: 01865 735 408
Fax: 01865 736 536
A country hotel that, with prior
arrangement, can cater for special
diets.

Wynncroft Hotel
2 Elmsleigh Park
Paignton
Devon TQ4 5AT
Tel: 01803 525 728
Fax: 01803 526 335
Website: www.wynncroft.co.uk
Caters mainly for gluten-free diets
but happy to discuss providing for
other diets.

Appendix 2
Useful Websites

INFORMATION

Many of the organisations listed in Appendix 1 have a website. Below are given general websites not listed in Appendix 1. Please note that these are given for your information only and should *not* be used to replace professional advice and treatment. Remember, too, that websites outside the UK will often use different terminology, weights and measures, trade names.

www.allallergy.net/allallergy/
Huge website created with the aim of pulling together all the other websites related to allergy

www.allerex.ca
This is *the* website for learning all about the EpiPen, including clinical information and how to give it correctly

www.allergicchild.com
A website created by parents of an allergic child. It aims to provide understanding and information as well as links to other websites and book information

www.allergies.about.com/
All about allergies, in user-friendly language

www.allergypack.com
Supplier of the Pen Pal, which is a versatile carry-bag for the EpiPen. The case is detachable from the strap and has Velcro straps for hooking onto bike handles etc., is insulated and shock resistant

www.allergyusa.com/
Allergy Care information and resources

www.anaphylaxis.org
Canadian equivalent of the UK Anaphylaxis Campaign

www.angelfire.com/mi/FAST
A non-commercial US site, run by a 19-year-old with a food allergy, devoted to educating the public about food allergy, with on-line discussion, support groups etc.

www.baronmoss.demon.co.uk
The website of Helen Stephenson, who has several food intolerances, including dairy products and eggs. Has excellent links to websites related to food allergies

www.choclat.com
Chocolate emporium: pareve speciality chocolates and other kosher confections for people needing dairy-free sweets

www.ctpa.org.uk
Site of the Cosmetic, Toiletry and Perfumery Association, giving the European Commission inventory of substances used in those products

www.darifree.comm
Non-dairy beverage that is potato based, and free from rice, soya and corn. Site has recipes and newsletter plus links to other sites

www.dg3.eudra.org
Gives the European Commission inventory of substances used in cosmetic, toiletry and perfumery products

www.dialspace.dial.pipex.com/town/park/gfm11/
A site devoted to dairy allergy and intolerance. Information, resources, articles and general help. Very informative

www.dspace.dial.pipex.com
Information for people allergic to milk or lactose-intolerant

www.efanet.org
Contains a teenagers' problem-page dedicated to providing teenagers with sound advice about asthma and other allergies, and a chat page

www.foodallergy.org
Website of the Food Allergy and Anaphylaxis Network (a non-profit-making US organisation), devoted to educating the public about food allergy and anaphylaxis, and advancing research. It publishes six newsletters a year and offers a range of resources

www.foodallergymatters.com
Useful site on all food allergy matters

www.glutenfree.com
US-based bakers with a wide range of products and recipe booklets – from stores and by mail order

www.golden.net/~zoniinc
Sales only. The Epi-belt will protect your emergency auto-injector in many conditions and, because you wear it, it provides quick easy access if required. Available as a single or double case attached to a belt or as a single or double holster

www.healthline.com/aa.htm
Allergy and Asthma magazine on-line

www.imaginefoods.com
Information about and sales of Rice Dream non-dairy beverages and desserts and soya milk

www.inside-story.com
Useful website with information on many aspects of allergy (including anaphylaxis), recipes, book list and links to related sites

www.lactoseintolerance.co.uk/
Website of the UK Allergy Network, for people allergic to milk and lactose intolerant

www.NoMilk.com
Information, recipes and advice for people with lactose maldigestion, milk allergy and casein intolerance

www.non-dairy.org
Comprehensive and informative site run by parents of children with allergy to dairy foods

www.nuttinwithnuts.com
A business (created by a sufferer) for people with a severe nut allergy and their families. On offer is education about anaphylaxis, patches, books and a neat EpiPen holder

www.organics.org
Plenty of information about organic products

www.peanutallergy.com
US site devoted to aspects of peanut allergy

www.protectube.com
Provide protective tubes for EpiPen. They are waterproof and buoyant, UV-protected and very durable. No more broken tubes or lost tops! Also carrying cases (Epi-Tote and Epi-Tote Twin) for the tubes

www.quorumallergy.com
Canadian company that supplies a variety of allergy-related products, including iron-on warning patches for clothes, knapsacks, etc. for children with food allergies. Also information about allergies and bibliography

www.theorganicshop.co.uk
For sales only. Over 600 organic products delivered to the door

www.veg.org/veg
Independent, definitive internet guide for vegetarians and vegans, with many valuable resources, recipes and links to related sites

www.veganvillage.co.uk
An excellent site with information on everything vegan

www.veggieheaven.com
The site to find vegetarian and vegan recipes, UK restaurant guide, nutritional guide, glossary, useful tips and links to related sites

BOOKS

The websites listed below (not mentioned elsewhere) give details of and/or produce information books and recipe books for allergy

www.amazon.com
On-line booksellers with a good range of recipe books and books on food allergy and intolerance

www.betterbaking.com/baker2/mock.html
For some books and a few small recipes

www.hallPublications.com
Books and other publications on food allergy and intolerance

www.nowbooks.co.uk
Online service for many booksellers in the UK and the USA

Appendix 3
Useful Publications

Below are listed publications that you might find helpful. In some cases they are published outside the UK but are available through your bookshop or local library or via the internet. Websites that have information about useful books are listed in Appendix 2.

INFORMATION BOOKS
Berlitz European Menu Reader. Berlitz Publishing, London, 1997.
Bird K, Farhall R, Rofe A, Whitlock J (Editors). *Animal-free Shopper*, 5th edition. Vegan Society, St Leonards on Sea, E Sussex, 2000 [animal-, dairy-, egg-free directory of products from food to cosmetics and cleaning agents]
Bremner M. *Genetic Engineering and You*. HarperCollins, London, 1999
Brostoff J, Gamlin L. *The Complete Guide to Food Allergy and Intolerance*. Bloomsbury, London, 1998
Clough J. *Allergies at your fingertips*. Class Publishing, London, 1997
Collins L. *Caring for Your Child with Severe Food Allergies: emotional support and practical advice from a parent who's been there*. Wiley, Chichester, 1999
Dibb S. *What the Label Doesn't Tell You*. Thorsons, London, 1998
Dibb S, Lobstein T. *GM Free: a shopper's guide to genetically modified foods*. Virgin, London: 1999
Dibb S, Mayer S. *Biotech – the next generation*. Food Commission, London, 2000
Duff S. *NHS Allergy Clinics*. British Society for Allergy and Clinical Immunology, Thames Ditton, Surrey, 1998 [reprint due in 2001]
Durham SR. *ABC of Allergies*. BMJ Books, London, 1998
Harvey J. *Managing Medicines in Schools*. Folens Publishers, Dublin, 1998
Joneja JV. *Dietary Management of Food Allergies and Intolerances: a comprehensive guide*, 2nd edn. J A Hall Publications, Burnaby BC, Canada, 1999 [also available from Merton Books]
Williams D, Williams A, Croker L. *Life-threatening Allergic Reactions: understanding and coping with anaphylaxis*. Piatkus, London, 1997

EATING OUT AND HOLIDAY ACCOMMODATION
Berlitz European Menu Reader. Berlitz Publishing, London, 1997
Bourke A (Editor) *Vegetarian Europe*. Vegetarian Guides, London
Bourke A, Gaynor P. *Vegetarian London*. Cruelty Free Living Publisher

Bourke A, Todd A. *Vegetarian Britain*, Vegetarian Guides, London
Bourke A, Todd A. *Vegetarian France*, Vegetarian Guides, London
Neiger E. *Food in Five Languages: an international menu guide*. Interlink
  Publishing Group, 1997 [in English, German, French, Italian, Spanish]
Rodger G. (Editor). *Vegan Passport*. Vegan Society, St Leonards on Sea, E Sussex,
  1996 [what vegans eat and don't eat, in 38 languages – useful for allergy to
  meat, fish, shellfish, milk, egg]
Vegan Society. *Vegan Travel Guide*. Vegan Society, St Leonards on Sea, E Sussex,
  [contains information on suitable places to stay and eat for vegans and those
  on egg-free, milk-free, fish/shellfish-free and meat-free diets, as well as
  details on hotels, B&Bs, guest houses, restaurants, cafés and tearooms, take-
  aways, pubs, wine bars and speciality holidays in Britain] Available from
  your local bookshop or direct from Vegetarian Guides Ltd, PO Box 2284,
  London W1A 5UH (www.vegetarianguides.co.uk)
Weitzel A. M. *Vegetarian Visitor: where to eat and stay in Britain*. Jon Carpenter
  Publishing, Chipping Norton, Oxon, 2000 [lists 300 establishments, many
  of which are used to catering for special diets]

CHILDREN'S BOOKS
The Diary of Cyril the Squirrel. Anaphylaxis Campaign, Fleet, Hants, 1996
  [about a squirrel who is allergic to nuts, the story is designed to help
  children come to terms with nut allergy]
Allie the Allergic Elephant. 1999. Available from Jungle Communications Inc.
  (Suite 3002500 North Circle Drive, Colorado Springs, CO 80919, USA),
  or from your local bookshop or via the internet if you quote the ISBN
  1–58628–050–3
Alexander the Elephant who couldn't eat Peanuts. Available from Allergy
  Essentials (59A Robertson Road, suite 148, Nepean Ontario, Ontario K2H
  5Y9, Canada)
Zevy A. *No Nuts for Me*. Tumbleweed Press (Unit 11, 401 Magnetic Drive,
  Downsview, Ontario M3J 3H9, Canada) [a story about how a little boy
  handles his food allergy at school]
Pre-schooler's Guide to Peanut Allergy. Ticketar Company, Vancouver BC V5N
  2E4, Canada (www.mcd.on.ca/ticketar/)
Troon H. *Aaron's Awful Allergies*. Kids Can Press, Toronto, Ontario, Canada,
  and Buffalo, NY, USA, 1998.

RECIPE BOOKS
Bronfman D, Bronfman R. *Calciyum! Delicious calcium-rich dairy-free vegetarian
  recipes*. Bromedia, Toronto, Ontario, 1998
Cole C. L. *Not Milk . . . Nut Milks*. Woodbridge Press, Santa Barbara CA, 1997

Crosthwaite F. *How to Eat Well again on a Wheat, Gluten and Dairy Free Diet.** Merton Books, Twickenham, 1997

Dumke N. M. *Easy Bread Making for Special Diets.* Adapt Books, Louisville CO, 1998

Emro R. *Bakin' Without Eggs.* St Martins Griffin, New York, 1999

Fenster C. *Special Diet Celebrations – no wheat, gluten, dairy or eggs.* Savory Palate Inc., Littleton CO, 1999

Graimes N. *The Vegan Cookbook.* Lorenz Books, London, 2000

Greer R. *Easy Wheat, Milk and Egg-free Cooking.* Thorsons, London, 2001

Hall P. H. *101 Fabulous Dairy-free Desserts Everyone Will Love.* Station Hill Openings, Barrytown NY, 1998

Kidder B. *The Milk-Free Kitchen.* Owl Books, New York, 1991

Lanza L, Morton L. *Totally Dairy-free Cooking.* William Morrow, New York, 1999

McCarty M. *Sweet and Natural: more than 120 naturally sweet and dairy-free desserts.* St Martin's Press, New York, 1999

Pannell M. *The Dairy-Free Cook Book.* Lorenz Books, London, 1999

Rawcliffe P, Ralph R. *The Gluten-free Diet.* Vermilion, London, 1997

Robertson R. *366 Simply Delicious Dairy-free Recipes.* Penguin, London, 1997

Stepaniak J. *The Uncheese Cookbook: creating amazing dairy-free substitutes and classic 'uncheese' dishes.* Book Publishing Co., Summertown TN, 1994

Wellington C. M. *Eating Well Milk-free.* Redpine Distributing ISBN 0-9699787-0-7

Wells D. *What Can I give Him Today?** Merton Books, Twickenham, 1998.

Zukin J. *Dairy-Free Cookbook.* Prima Health, Rocklin CA, 1998

Zukin J. *Raising Your Child Without Milk: reassuring advice and recipes for parents of lactose-intolerant and milk-allergic children.* Prima Publishing, Rocklin CA, 1995.

* Details of these and other allergy recipe books are available from Action Against Allergy (AAA)

LEAFLETS

Useful leaflets are available from the head offices of most food manufacturers and retailers (supermarkets) and the health promotion department of your local health authority, as well as from the following (contact details in the 'Useful addresses' appendix):

Action Against Allergy
Anaphylaxis Campaign
British Allergy Foundation
EFA (European Federation of Asthma and Allergy Associations)
MAFF Consumer Helpline 0645 556 000
UCB Institute of Allergy

BOOKLETS

Adverse Reactions to Food. European Federation of Asthma and Allergy
    Associations (EFA), 1997; also available on ww.astmafonds.nl/
    astmafonds/brochure/allergie.phtml
Adverse Reactions to Foods. British Nutrition Foundation, London, 1995
Nut Allergy: it's not a game of chance. Anaphylaxis Campaign, Fleet, Hants,
    1999 [aimed specifically at young people]
Health Advice for Travellers. Department of Health, London, 2000 (copies from
    0800 555 777)
Fowler K, Smithers F. *The L-Plate Vegan.* Viva!, Brighton, 1999 [excellent
    product information on foods free from dairy, eggs, animals]

MAGAZINES

Allergy News available free to members of the British Allergy Foundation, or
    can be bought from newsagents and some supermarkets
The Food Magazine, a good quarterly magazine published by the Food
    Commission
Also available are quarterly newsletters for members of Action Against Allergy
    and the Anaphylaxis Campaign.

REPORTS

COT, for the Department of Health. *Peanut Allergy.* Department of Health,
    London, 1998
Department for Education and Employment. *Supporting Pupils with Medical
    Needs in School.* Department of Health, London, 1996
Department for Education and Employment. *Supporting Pupils with Medical
    Needs: a good practice guide.* Department of Health, London, 1996
Dibb S, Fitzpatrick M. *Soya Infant Formula: the health concerns.* Food
    Commission, London, 1998
European Allergy White Paper: *Allergic Diseases as a Public Health Problem.* UCB
    Institute of Allergy, Watford, Herts, 1997
European Allergy White Paper – *Update.* UCB Institute of Allergy, Watford,
    Herts, 1999
Guidance Notes: *Labelling of Food containing Genetically Modified Soya or Maize.*
    Ministry of Agriculture, Fisheries and Food, London, 1999

VIDEOS

Learning to Live with Anaphylaxis An information video on anaphylaxis for parents, schools, child carers and health professionals. Anaphylaxis Campaign, London*

Action for Anaphylaxis Role-play of a child having an anaphylactic reaction at school and the action taken based on training received by the school staff. Anaphylaxis Campaign, London*

A Race Against Time About the Anapen and its use during anaphylaxis. Available free from Allerayde*

*Contact details in Appendix 1

Index

Note: Page numbers in *italics* indicate tables or illustrations; those in **bold** indicate emergency action; those with *g* refer to the glossary.

Have you found *Food Allergies: Enjoying Life with a Severe Food Allergy* useful and practical? If so, you may be interested in other books from Class Publishing.

Allergies at your fingertips

Dr Joanne Clough   £14.99

Sensible, practical advice on allergies from an experienced medical expert. Dr Clough answers over 300 real questions from people with allergies and their families, giving you advice you can trust.

'An excellent book which deserves to be on the bookshelf of every family.'
Dr Csaba Rusznak, Medical and Scientific Director, British Allergy Foundation

Asthma at your fingertips

NEW THIRD EDITION!   £14.99

Dr Mark Levy, Professor Sean Hilton and Greta Barnes MBE

This book shows you how to keep your asthma – or your family's asthma – under control, making it easier to live a full, happy and healthy life.

'This book gives you the knowledge. Don't limit yourself.'
Adrian Moorhouse MBE, Olympic Gold Medallist

Eczema and your child

Dr Tim Mitchell, Dr David Paige and Karen Spowart   £11.99

This practical and medically accurate handbook will guide you through the maze of old wives' tales, unscientific advice and outdated treatments.

Psoriasis at your fingertips

Dr Tim Mitchell and Rebecca Penzer
NEW!   £14.99

Packed full of practical information on the day-to-day management of psoriasis. This essential manual tells you about the various treatments available, helping you to discover which work best for you, and giving you effective self-help routines.

High blood pressure at your fingertips

NEW SECOND EDITION!   £14.99

Dr Julian Tudor Hart with Dr Tom Fahey

The authors use all their years of experience as blood pressure experts to answer your questions on high blood pressure.

'Readable and comprehensive information.'
Dr Sylvia McLaughlan, Director General, The Stroke Association

Diabetes at your fingertips

FOURTH EDITION!   £14.99

Professor Peter Sonksen, Dr Charles Fox and Sister Sue Judd

461 questions on diabetes are answered clearly and accurately – the ideal reference book for everyone with diabetes.

Heart health at your fingertips

NEW SECOND EDITION!   £14.99

Dr Graham Jackson

This practical handbook, written by a leading cardiologist, answers all your questions about heart conditions.

'Contains the answers the doctor wishes he had given if only he'd had the time'
Dr Thomas Stuttaford, The Times

PRIORITY ORDER FORM

Cut out or photocopy this form and send it (*post free in the UK*) to:

**Class Publishing Priority Service,
FREEPOST (PAM 6219) Plymouth PL6 7ZZ
Tel: (01752) 202301   Fax: (01752) 202333**

Please send me urgently (*tick boxes below*)

*Post included
price per copy
(UK only)*

☐	**Food Allergies: Enjoying life with a severe food allergy** (ISBN 1 859590 39 X)	£17.99
☐	**Allergies at your fingertips** (ISBN 1 872362 52 4)	£17.99
☐	**Asthma at your fingertips** (ISBN 1 85959 006 3)	£17.99
☐	**Eczema and your child: A parent's guide** (ISBN 1 872362 86 9)	£14.99
☐	**Psoriasis at your fingertips** (ISBN 1 872362 99 0)	£17.99
☐	**High blood pressure at your fingertips** (ISBN 1 872362 81 8)	£17.99
☐	**Diabetes at your fingertips** (ISBN 1 872362 79 6)	£17.99
☐	**Heart health at your fingertips** (ISBN 1 85959 009 8)	£17.99
	TOTAL	_____

Easy ways to pay

Cheque: I enclose a cheque payable to Class Publishing for £ _____

Credit card: Please debit my ☐ Access ☐ Visa ☐ Amex ☐ Switch

Number _____ Expiry date _____ / _____

Name _____

My address for delivery is _____

_____

Town _____ County _____ Postcode _____

Telephone number (*in case of query*) _____

Credit card billing address if different from above _____

_____

Town _____ County _____ Postcode _____

*Class Publishing's guarantee: Remember that if, for any reason, you are not satisfied with these books,
we will refund all your money, without any questions asked. Prices and VAT rates may be altered
for reasons beyond our control.*